Psychiatric Manifestations of Neurotoxins

Editors

DANIEL E. RUSYNIAK
MICHAEL R. DOBBS

PSYCHIATRIC CLINICS OF NORTH AMERICA

www.psych.theclinics.com

June 2013 • Volume 36 • Number 2

ELSEVIER

1600 John F. Kennedy Boulevard ● Suite 1800 ● Philadelphia, Pennsylvania, 19103-2899

http://www.theclinics.com

PSYCHIATRIC CLINICS OF NORTH AMERICA Volume 36, Number 2
June 2013 ISSN 0193-953X, ISBN-13: 978-1-4557-7146-2

Editor: Joanne Husovski
Developmental Editor: Donald Mumford

Psychiatric Clinics of North America (ISSN 0193-953X) is published quarterly by Elsevier Inc., 360 Park Avenue South, New York, NY 10010-1710. Months of issue are March, June, September, and December. Business and Editorial Offices: 1600 John F. Kennedy Blvd., Suite 1800, Philadelphia, PA 19103-2899. Periodicals postage paid at New York, NY and additional mailing offices. Subscription prices are $286.00 per year (US individuals), $524.00 per year (US institutions), $141.00 per year (US students/residents), $347.00 per year (Canadian individuals), $651.00 per year (Canadian Institutions), $431.00 per year (foreign individuals), $651.00 per year (foreign institutions), and $210.00 per year (international & Canadian students/residents). Foreign air speed delivery is included in all *Clinics'* subscription prices. All prices are subject to change without notice. **POSTMASTER:** Send address changes to *Psychiatric Clinics of North America*, Elsevier Health Sciences Division, Subscription Customer Service, 3251 Riverport Lane, Maryland Heights, MO 63043. Customer Service: 1-800-654-2452 (US). From outside the United States, call 1-314-447-8871. Fax: 1-314-447-8029. E-mail: journalscustomerservice-usa@elsevier.com (for print support) and journalsonlinesupport-usa@elsevier.com (for online support).

Reprints. For copies of 100 or more, of articles in this publication, please contact the Commercial Reprints Department, Elsevier Inc., 360 Park Avenue South, New York, New York 10010-1710. Tel.: (212) 633-3813, Fax: (212) 462-1935, E-mail: reprints@elsevier.com.

Psychiatric Clinics of North America is covered in *MEDLINE/PubMed (Index Medicus)*, *Current Contents/Social and Behavioral Sciences, Social Science Citation Index, Embase/Excerpta Medica,* and PsycINFO.

Printed and bound by CPI Group (UK) Ltd, Croydon, CR0 4YY

Transferred to digital print 2013

Contributors

EDITORS

DANIEL E. RUSYNIAK, MD
Associate Professor of Emergency Medicine, Adjunct Associate Professor of Pharmacology, Toxicology, and Clinical Neurology, Department of Emergency Medicine, Indiana University School of Medicine, Indianapolis, Indiana

MICHAEL R. DOBBS, MD
Department of Neurology, University of Kentucky College of Medicine, Lexington, Kentucky

AUTHORS

J. DAVE BARRY, MD
Director, Emergency Medicine Residency Program; Department of Emergency Medicine, Naval Medical Center Portsmouth, Portsmouth, Virginia; Assistant Professor of Military and Emergency Medicine, Uniformed Services University of the Health Sciences, Bethesda, Maryland

CHRISTOPHER M. FILLEY, MD
Departments of Neurology and Psychiatry, University of Colorado School of Medicine; Denver Veterans Affairs Medical Center, Aurora, Colorado

DONG Y. HAN, PsyD
Neuropsychology Section, Department of Neurology, University of Kentucky, Lexington, Kentucky

BRYAN S. JUDGE, MD
Associate Program Director, Grand Rapids Medical Education Partners/Michigan State University Emergency Medicine Residency; Associate Professor, Division of Emergency Medicine, Michigan State University College of Human Medicine; Spectrum Health-Toxicology Services, Grand Rapids, Michigan

HANI A. KUSHLAF, MB, BCh
Assistant Professor of Neurology and Pathology, Department of Neurology, University of Cincinnati, Cincinnati, Ohio

LISA H. MASON, MS
Neuropsychology Section, Department of Neurology, University of Kentucky, Lexington, Kentucky

MELISSA J. MATHEWS, PhD
Neuropsychology Section, Department of Neurology, University of Kentucky, Lexington, Kentucky

LANDEN L. RENTMEESTER, MD
Assistant Clinical Instructor, Division of Emergency Medicine, Michigan State University College of Human Medicine; Resident Physician, Grand Rapids Medical Education Partners/Michigan State University Emergency Medicine Residency, Grand Rapids, Michigan

DANIEL E. RUSYNIAK, MD
Associate Professor of Emergency Medicine, Adjunct Associate Professor of Pharmacology, Toxicology, and Clinical Neurology, Department of Emergency Medicine, Indiana University School of Medicine, Indianapolis, Indiana

LAURA M. TORMOEHLEN, MD
Assistant Professor of Clinical Neurology, Departments of Neurology and Emergency Medicine, Indiana University School of Medicine, Indianapolis, Indiana

BRANDON K. WILLS, DO, MS
Director, Medical Toxicology Fellowship, Virginia Commonwealth University Medical Center; Assistant Professor, Department of Emergency Medicine, Virginia Commonwealth University Health Center; Associated Medical Director, Virginia Poison Center, Richmond, Virginia

Contents

> The goal of this review is to provide guidelines for evaluating psychiatric and mood changes that result from neurotoxicity. Mood changes that are often seen to varying degrees in neurotoxicity include increased anxiety, depression, irritability, impulsiveness, and psychosis. Some common agents that induce neurotoxicity include drugs, heavy metals, and organophosphates with presentations varying somewhat depending upon the mechanism of toxicity. The authors discuss in detail psychiatric assessment for patients with suspected of having neurotoxicologic syndrome.

> Psychiatrists in practice encounter patients abusing alcohol and street drugs such as cocaine that can lead to toxic myopathies or neuropathies. Psychiatrists also encounter patients with neuropsychiatric systemic lupus erythematosus who are treated with myotoxic medications (e.g., Hydroxychloroquine). Thus a well-rounded knowledge of toxic myopathies and neuropathies is extremely useful. The differential diagnosis of toxic myopathies and neuropathies is expanding rapidly and practical knowledge of these entities is becoming important.

> This article is intended for clinicians treating neurotoxic emergencies. Presented are causative agents of neurotoxic emergencies, many of which are easily mistaken for acute psychiatric disorders. Understanding the wide variety of agents responsible for neurotoxic emergencies and the neurotransmitter interactions involved will help the psychiatrist identify and treat this challenging population.

> Treating patients with psychiatric problems can present numerous challenges for clinicians. The deliberate self-ingestion of antidepressants is one such challenge frequently encountered in hospitals throughout the United States. This review focuses on 1) the classes of antidepressants, their pharmacologic properties, and some of the proposed mechanism(s) for antidepressant overdose-induced seizures; 2) the evidence for seizures caused by antidepressants in overdose; 3) management strategies for

PSYCHIATRIC CLINICS OF NORTH AMERICA

RELATED INTEREST

Neurotoxicology and Teratology
March—April 2012 (Vol. 34, No. 2)
**Behavioral Toxicology of Cognition: Extrapolation from Experimental Animal
Models to Humans: Behavioral Toxicology Symposium Overview**
Merle G. Paule, Leonard Green, Joel Myerson, et al.

**DOWNLOAD
Free App!**

Review Articles
THE CLINICS

NOW AVAILABLE FOR YOUR iPhone and iPad

Preface

Neurotoxicology: The Ties that Bind Us

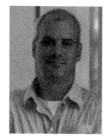 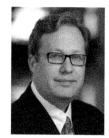

Daniel E. Rusyniak, MD   Michael R. Dobbs, MD
                    Editors

We are honored to be asked to publish in *Psychiatric Clinics of North America* many of the articles on neurotoxicology from our edition of *Neurologic Clinics*. We believe these articles, along with one from the Neuropsychiatric issue edited by Dr Silvia Riggio, as well as several new articles are a natural fit for this issue, as the specialties of Psychiatry, Neurology, and Medical Toxicology are, in many ways, inseparable.

As highlighted in these articles, there are numerous examples in which changes in personality, behavior, and emotion are clinical findings of neurotoxicity: psychosis after chronic methamphetamine abuse (see article by Rusyniak); disinhibited behaviors in patients with toxin-induced leukoenchephalopathies (see article by Tormoehlen and Filley); and CNS depression, agitation, aggression (see article by Lane, Kjome, and Moeller) and confusion in a variety of neurotoxic emergencies (see article by Barry and Willis). The myriad of presentations after neurotoxic exposures highlight the importance of having toxins in the differential of any patient presenting with a psychiatric complaint and the need for the development of better and more specific testing (see article by Han et al). In addition to toxins causing psychiatric symptoms, the most common medical problems in patients admitted for drug overdose are psychiatric. This is due, in part, to the high rates of drug abuse in patients with mental illnesses, their risk for self harm, and the toxicity of the drugs they take to treat mental illness (eg, the most common cause of drug-induced seizures are antidepressants [see article by Judge and Rentmeester]). Last, the trigger of many neurologic and mental illnesses may be environmental exposures to toxins like pesticides and heavy metals (see articles by Jett and Jang and Hoffman) or even household products like denture paste (see article by Kaushlaf). Unfortunately, causal associations between these exposures and mental disorders are still lacking, leading some patients to search for cures in untested and unconventional treatments such as metal chelation (see article by Jang and Hoffman).

Psychiatr Clin N Am 36 (2013) ix–x
http://dx.doi.org/10.1016/j.psc.2013.02.007
0193-953X/13/$ – see front matter © 2013 Published by Elsevier Inc.

psych.theclinics.com

As indicated by these articles, the specialties of Medical Toxicology, Psychiatry, and Neurology are closely linked by drugs and toxins. Therefore, we should not view neurotoxicology as a niche or separate specialty, but rather as a medical field requiring shared knowledge and expertise. Better interprofessional communication and collaboration among our specialties will ultimately improve our understanding of neurotoxins, and our patients will be the better for it.

Daniel E. Rusyniak, MD
Department of Emergency Medicine
Indiana University School of Medicine
1050 Wishard Boulevard, Room 2200
Indianapolis, IN 46202, USA

Michael R. Dobbs, MD
Department of Neurology
University of Kentucky College of Medicine
740 South Limestone Street
Wing D, KY Clinic
Lexington, KY 40536, USA

E-mail addresses:
drusynia@iupui.edu (D.E. Rusyniak)
mrdobb0@uky.edu (M.R. Dobbs)

Neuropsychiatric Symptom Assessments in Toxic Exposure

Lisa H. Mason, MS, Melissa J. Mathews, PhD, Dong Y. Han, PsyD*

KEYWORDS

- Toxin • Neurotoxin • Toxic exposure • Neuropsychiatric assessment

KEY POINTS

- Typical manifestations of neurotoxicity include changes in cognitive function, neurologic function, mood, and psychiatric disturbances.
- Psychiatric changes often seen to varying degrees in neurotoxicity include increased anxiety, depression, irritability, impulsiveness, and psychosis.
- Among common agents that induce neurotoxicity are drugs, heavy metals, and organophosphates.
- A multidisciplinary approach involving psychiatry, neurology, neuropsychology, and other appropriate providers is likely the best approach to patient care.

BEHAVIORAL MANIFESTATIONS OF NEUROTOXICITY

Neurotoxicity is the disruption of the nervous system resulting from exposure to environmental toxins. Typical manifestations include changes in cognitive function and the development of neurodegenerative memory disorders (for a review, see Han and colleagues[1] and Caban-Holt and colleagues[2]), changes in neurologic function, and mood/psychiatric disturbances. This article provides guidelines for evaluating psychiatric and mood changes that result from neurotoxicity. Mood changes that are often seen to varying degrees in neurotoxicity include increased anxiety, depression, irritability, impulsiveness, and psychosis. Some common agents that induce neurotoxicity include drugs, heavy metals, and organophosphates, with presentations varying depending on the mechanism of toxicity.

Drugs

One drug commonly used to treat bipolar mania is lithium. Acute toxicity involves primarily physical symptoms such as gastrointestinal upset (ie, nausea, vomiting,

Neuropsychology Section, Department of Neurology, University of Kentucky, 740 South Limestone Street, Suite L445, Lexington, KY 40536-0284, USA
* Corresponding author. Department of Neurology, University of Kentucky College of Medicine, 740 South Limestone Street, Suite L445, Lexington, KY 40536-0284.
E-mail address: d.han@uky.edu

Psychiatr Clin N Am 36 (2013) 201–208
http://dx.doi.org/10.1016/j.psc.2013.02.001
0193-953X/13/$ – see front matter © 2013 Elsevier Inc. All rights reserved.

psych.theclinics.com

diarrhea), dizziness, weakness, and potentially seizures, coma, ataxia, and tremor depending on the dose. However, chronic lithium toxicity typically presents with kidney and nervous system damage, including psychosis. Episodes of hypomania[3] and Capgras syndrome[4] have also been reported. Local anesthetics such as lidocaine may also have adverse psychiatric side effects such as euphoria, psychosis, or agitation.[5] In a study of 20 patients, Gil-Gouveia and Goadsby[5] found that 75% of their patients had psychiatric sequelae after receiving lidocaine for headache. Symptoms included dysphoria, depressive symptoms, depressive mood concurrent with paranoia, and agitation concurrent with both auditory and visual hallucinations. Their review of the literature yielded a wide range of psychiatric events (1.8%–100%). Antiretroviral therapies used to treat human immunodeficiency virus/acquired immunodeficiency syndrome have also been thought to pose a risk for central nervous system toxicity[6]; however, some studies have found beneficial effects for both cognition and mood using zidovudine (AZT).[7]

Polydrug use including marijuana and ecstasy has been linked to impulsivity, emotional lability, aggression, anxiety, and depression.[8–12] Marijuana and opioid users self-reported higher levels of trait anxiety and depression. Inhalants were associated with higher levels of trait anxiety, apathy, disinhibition, and executive dysfunction.[13]

Heavy Metals

Heavy metals include arsenic, lead, mercury, and manganese among many others. Toxicity from these elements may manifest acutely or chronically and symptom presentation may vary accordingly. Acute toxicity is typically characterized by rapid onset and numerous gastrointestinal symptoms (eg, nausea, vomiting) along with headaches and changes in cognition and motor skills. However, long-term exposure may result in clear neurodegeneration that mimics neurodegenerative diseases such as Parkinson disease. Psychiatric manifestations of heavy metal neurotoxicity may occur after even small exposures. For example, modest exposure to lead was positively correlated with phobic anxiety.[14]

Manganese is a heavy metal that is frequently found in many industrial occupations such as mining, welding, and working with fertilizers. Symptoms may vary according to level of exposure to manganese. Manganese exposure through working at a ferroalloy plant was measured in terms of cumulated exposure indices (CEI) accounting for each worker's level of exposure to manganese-containing dust per year of employment. When examined as groups with high, medium, and low exposure, those with the greatest exposure were significantly higher on self-report measures of somatization, depression, anxiety, and hostility compared with nonexposed controls. Participants in the middle group reported significantly more depression and anxiety than controls, whereas those in the lowest exposure group did not differ on any psychiatric/mood indices.[15] Furthermore, symptom presentation may vary according to whether the toxicity is acute or chronic. Acute onset may present with neurologic or psychotic disturbances. Acute psychosis has been described as including excitability, agitation, and hallucinations or delusions. Irritability and mild conduct and behavior problems have also been noted. Insidious onset is variable in its presentation and may include neurologic abnormalities, neuropsychiatric abnormalities, or fatigue, slowed thought processes, and poor concentration. Generalized weakness, fatigue, and sleep disturbance are some early symptoms seen in insidious onset.[16] Manganese toxicity also frequently presents with similar symptoms to idiopathic Parkinson disease and may be difficult to differentiate from this neurodegenerative disease.[17,18] Psychiatric symptoms in manganese toxicity may present either before or concurrently with motor signs typical of Parkinson disease (ie, rigidity, bradykinesia, and balance and gait difficulties) and include compulsive behavior, emotional instability, and psychotic symptoms like hallucinations.[18,19]

Organophosphates and Organic Solvents

Organophosphates are found in many daily household products such as pesticides and solvents; however, they are known to have toxic effects on humans. Acute toxic effects are likely related to excess acetylcholine caused by cholinesterase inhibition.[20,21] Common psychiatric manifestations of acute organophosphate exposure include anxiety, irritability, and depression. Regarding chronic effects of organophosphate toxicity, confusion, anxiety, and depression have also been observed.[21–23] For example, Ross and colleagues[23] found that low-level exposure resulted in significantly greater anxiety and depression in exposed groups (40%) compared with controls (23%). Morrow and colleagues[24] also found that 50% of their participants who had been exposed to organic solvents met established mood disorder criteria using a structured clinical interview.

PSYCHIATRIC ASSESSMENT FOR PATIENTS WITH NEUROTOXICOLOGIC SYNDROME

Formal assessment of psychiatric symptoms in persons suspected to have neurotoxicologic syndrome should focus on changes in mood, evaluation of psychotic symptoms, and frontal executive dysfunction. No widely accepted specific guideline exists at this time. However, given that anxiety and depression are common psychiatric manifestations regardless of the toxin, it may be helpful to administer structured self-report measures in conjunction with careful clinical evaluation of symptoms. Ascertaining the degree to which the current level of anxiety and depression differ from the baseline before toxin exposure may provide a clue to whether symptoms are related to neurotoxicity. Psychosis may be present when the neurotoxicologic syndrome is caused by drug side effects or heavy metal exposure. Thus, persons with known exposure to these elements should be evaluated for psychosis. In contrast, in persons presenting with acute psychosis, drug intoxication or exposure to heavy metals should also be considered as a rule-out diagnosis. Regarding frontal dysexecutive syndrome, numerous studies reported observations of irritability, impulsivity, and emotional lability, aggression, and executive dysfunction. Thus, structured assessment of frontal behaviors in addition to clinical evaluation of personality changes in terms of hostility, agitation, impulsivity, and emotional instability provides a valuable addition to the evaluation of psychiatric symptoms.

This article addresses the following assessments, ranging from self-assessment to structured interview:

- Brief Symptom Inventory (BSI)
- Symptom Checklist-90-Revised (SCL-90-R)
- Minnesota Multiphasic Personality Inventory-2 (MMPI-2)
- Profile of Mood Scale 2nd Edition (POMS 2)
- Beck Depression Inventory 2nd Edition (BDI-II)
- Beck Anxiety Inventory (BAI)
- Structured Clinical Interview for Diagnostic and Statistical Manual of Mental Disorders, Fourth Edition (DSM-IV) Disorders (SCID-I)

Multisymptom Self-report Measures

BSI

The BSI[25] is a brief self-report inventory that may be administered in a paper-and-pencil fashion or via computer. Completion time is approximately 8 to 10 minutes.

The BSI is appropriate for use with individuals aged 13 years or older who have at least a sixth grade reading level. The BSI provides scores for 9 scales:

1. Somatization
2. Obsessive-compulsive
3. Interpersonal sensitivity
4. Depression
5. Anxiety
6. Hostility
7. Phobic anxiety
8. Paranoid ideation
9. Psychoticism

In addition, the BSI provides 3 global indices, for:

1. Overall distress level
2. Intensity of symptoms
3. Number of self-reported items

As such, the BSI may be especially useful for determining intensity of distress levels along with symptom presentation for a variety of psychiatric disturbances.

SCL-90-R

The SCL-90-R[26] shares many common features with the BSI, including reading level, patient age, and intended use to determine intensity and presence of psychiatric symptoms. The SCL-90-R also contains the aforementioned 9 symptom dimension scales and 3 global indices. However, the SCL-90-R is longer, consisting of 90 items and requiring approximately 12 to 15 minutes for administration. Benefits of this expanded self-report measure include expanded symptom assessment and identification of potential psychiatric problems before acute onset. The SCL-90-R may also be used to track progress over time, enabling appropriate treatment monitoring and guidance.

MMPI-2

The MMPI-2[27] is a longer and more comprehensive assessment of psychiatric disorders. Administration time ranges from 60 to 90 minutes. However, required reading level is lower than the aforementioned tests at a minimum of the fifth grade. One benefit of the MMPI-2 is the presence of validity scales that detect response inconsistency, endorsement of infrequent symptoms, overly positive self-presentation, and exaggeration of symptoms. The MMPI-2 produces 9 clinical scale scores:

1. Hypochondriasis
2. Depression
3. Hysteria
4. Psychopathic deviance
5. Masculinity-femininity
6. Paranoia
7. Psychasthenia
8. Schizophrenia
9. Hypomania

An additional scale assesses social introversion and various clinical subscales offer more detailed information regarding symptom type and severity. Thus, the MMPI-2 is appropriate for use in detecting the presence of anxiety, depression, psychosis, and other psychiatric symptoms. Validity scale inclusion makes the MMPI-2 especially appropriate when clinicians suspect effort levels, such as when working with compensation-seeking individuals.

POMS 2

The POMS 2[28] is a brief self-report inventory that assesses mood states of individuals 13 years of age or older. A new youth version is also available for the assessment of individuals aged 13 to 17 years. The POMS 2 includes 7 subscales that assess for both transient and chronic mood states in the following domains:

1. Anger-hostility
2. Confusion-bewilderment
3. Depression-dejection
4. Fatigue-inertia
5. Tension-anxiety
6. Vigor-activity
7. Friendliness

Both a long form and a short form are available, with administration times of 10 to 15 minutes and 5 to 10 minutes, respectively.

Self-report Depression Measure

Beck Depression Inventory-II (BDI-II)

The BDI-II[29] is a commonly used self-report depression inventory, appropriate for use with individuals aged 13 to 80 years. The BDI-II is brief, consisting of 21 items that assess the intensity of depression symptoms as defined by DSM-IV criteria. Each item consists of a symptom followed by descriptor items arranged from least to most severe. The person being evaluated is asked to endorse symptom levels that they have experienced in the past 2 weeks. Total scores correspond with the following interpretive categories of depressive symptoms:

- Minimal
- Mild
- Moderate
- Severe

The BDI-II is intended for use as a screening tool, but may also be used to track symptoms over time.

Self-report Anxiety Measure

BAI

The BAI[30] is a commonly used self-report anxiety inventory, appropriate for use with individuals aged 17 to 80 years. The BAI is brief (5–10 minutes administration time), consisting of 21 items that assess the intensity of anxiety symptoms. The BAI is a widely used screening tool, and has been shown to discriminate between clinically anxious and nonanxious individuals. Items consist of symptom descriptions and response columns ranging from not at all to severely. Persons being evaluated are asked to respond to each item describing presence and severity of symptoms. Total scores correspond with the following interpretive categories: minimal, mild, moderate, or severe anxiety symptoms.

Structured Interview

SCID-I

The SCID-I[31] is a clinician administered semistructured interview that aids in diagnosis formulation of DSM-IV T text revision (DSM-IV-TR) diagnoses. The SCID-I consists of 9 diagnostic modules that correspond with DSM-IV-TR diagnoses. However, the clinician can choose to skip modules to concentrate on suspected diagnoses, such as anxiety, depression, or psychosis. SCID-I administration times range depending on the number of administered modules and depth/breadth of symptom coverage (may be up to 2 hours). Advantages include expanded reports of symptoms and symptom severity, increased rapport building, and in-depth assessment of an individual's symptoms.

SUMMARY

Neurotoxic exposure can result in a variety of psychiatric sequelae, including manifestations of anxiety, depression, and psychotic symptoms (**Table 1**). Thus, appropriate psychiatric care requires assessment of multiple psychiatric domains and is best accomplished through the use of a multiscale inventory or the combination of multiple symptom assessment tools. Further, neurotoxic exposure may cause symptoms that are best cared for by additional treatment providers. A multidisciplinary approach involving psychiatry, neurology, neuropsychology, and other appropriate

Table 1 Neurotoxins and potential psychiatric manifestations or sequelae	
Neurotoxin	**Psychiatric Manifestations**
Lithium	Acute: physical symptoms Chronic: psychosis, hypomania, Capgras syndrome
Lidocaine	Euphoria, psychosis, agitation, dysphoria, depressive symptoms, depressive mood with paranoia, hallucinations
Antiretroviral therapies AZT	Risk for central nervous system toxicity Potential benefit for cognition and mood
Polydrug: marijuana and ecstasy	Depression, impulsivity, aggression, anxiety, emotional lability
Heavy metals	Acute: physical plus cognition and motor skill decline. Neurologic or psychotic disturbances, including excitability, agitation, and hallucinations or delusions. Irritability and mild conduct and behavior problems Chronic: neurodegeneration mimicking Parkinson disease. Variable presentation may include neurologic abnormalities, neuropsychiatric abnormalities, or fatigue, slowed thought processes, and poor concentration. Early symptoms are generalized weakness, fatigue, and sleep disturbance
Lead	Low exposure: correlated with phobic anxiety
Manganese	Low exposure: no correlation with psychiatric or mood disturbances Medium exposure: higher depression and anxiety compared with nonexposed High exposure: higher somatization, depression, anxiety, and hostility compared with nonexposed
Organophosphates	Acute: anxiety, irritability, depression Chronic: confusion, anxiety, depression

providers is likely the best approach to patient care. This team approach, along with sensitivity to the patient's distress, is likely to enhance treatment quality and patient recovery.

REFERENCES

1. Han DY, Hoelzle JB, Dennis BC, et al. A brief review of cognitive assessment in neurotoxicology. Neurol Clin 2011;29(3):581–90.
2. Caban-Holt A, Mattingly M, Cooper G, et al. Neurodegenerative memory disorders: a potential role of environmental toxins. Neurol Clin 2005;23(2):485–521.
3. Wright P, Seth R. Lithium toxicity, hypomania and leukocytosis with fluoxetine. Ir J Psychol Med 1992;9(1):59–60.
4. Nagasawa H, Hayashi H, Otani K. Capgras syndrome occurring in lithium toxicity. Clin Neuropharmacol 2012;35(4):204.
5. Gil-Gouveia R, Goadsby PJ. Neuropsychiatric side-effects of lidocaine: examples from the treatment of headache and a review. Cephalalgia 2009;29(5):496–508.
6. Carr A, Cooper DA. Adverse effects of antiretroviral therapy. Lancet 2000; 356(9239):1423–30.
7. Schmitt FA, Bigley JW, McKinnis R, et al. Neuropsychological outcome of zidovudine (AZT) Treatment of patients with AIDS and AIDS-related complex. N Engl J Med 1988;319(24):1573–8.
8. Gouzoulis-Mayfrank E, Daumann J. Neurotoxicity of methylenedioxyamphetamines (MDMA; ecstasy) in humans: how strong is the evidence for persistent brain damage? Addiction 2006;101(3):348–61.
9. Morgan MJ. Recreational use of "Ecstasy" (MDMA) is associated with elevated impulsivity. Neuropsychopharmacology 1998;19(4):252–64.
10. Daumann J, Pelz S, Becker S, et al. Psychological profile of abstinent recreational Ecstasy (MDMA) users and significance of concomitant cannabis use. Hum Psychopharmacol 2001;16(8):627–33.
11. MacInnes N, Handley SL, Harding GF. Former chronic methylenedioxymethamphetamine (MDMA or ecstasy) users report mild depressive symptoms. J Psychopharmacol 2001;15(3):181–6.
12. McCardle K, Luebbers S, Carter JD, et al. Chronic MDMA (ecstasy) use, cognition and mood. Psychopharmacology 2004;173(3–4):434–9.
13. Medina KL, Shear PK. Anxiety, depression, and behavioral symptoms of executive dysfunction in ecstasy users: contributions of polydrug use. Drug Alcohol Depend 2007;87(2–3):303–11.
14. Rhodes D, Spiro A, Aro A, et al. Relationship to bone and blood lead levels to psychiatric symptoms: the normative aging study. J Occup Environ Med 2003; 45(11):1144–51.
15. Bouchard M, Mergler D, Baldwin M, et al. Neuropsychiatric symptoms and past manganese exposure in a ferro-alloy plant. Neurotoxicology 2007;28(2):290–7.
16. Naby SA, Hassanein M. Neuropsychiatric manifestations of chronic manganese poisoning. J Neurol Neurosurg Psychiatr 1965;28:282.
17. Racette BA, Perlmutter JS. Welding-related parkinsonism: clinical features, treatment, and pathophysiology [reply]. Neurology 2001;57(9):1739.
18. Huang CC, Chu NS, Lu CS, et al. Chronic manganese intoxication. Arch Neurol 1989;46(10):1104–6.
19. Barceloux DG. Manganese. J Toxicol Clin Toxicol 1999;37(2):293–307.
20. Gallo MA, Lawryk NJ. Organic phosphorus pesticides. San Diego (CA): Academic Press; 1991.

21. Mearns J, Dunn J, Leeshaley PR. Psychological effects of organophosphate pesticides - a review and call for research by psychologists. J Clin Psychol 1994;50(2):286–94.
22. Colosio C, Tiramani M, Maroni M. Neurobehavioral effects of pesticides: state of the art. Neurotoxicology 2003;24(4–5):577–91.
23. Ross SJ, Brewin CR, Curran HV, et al. Neuropsychological and psychiatric functioning in sheep farmers exposed to low levels of organophosphate pesticides. Neurotoxicol Teratol 2010;32(4):452–9.
24. Morrow LA, Stein L, Bagovich GR, et al. Neuropsychological assessment, depression, and past exposure to organic solvents. Appl Neuropsychol 2001;8: 65–73.
25. Derogatis LR, Melisaratos N. The brief symptom inventory - an introductory report. Psychol Med 1983;13(3):595–605.
26. Derogatis LR. SCL-90-R, administration, scoring, and procedures. Manual for the (revised) version. Baltimore (MD): John Hopkins University School of Medicine; 1977.
27. Butcher JN, Dahlstrom WG, Graham JR, et al. Manual for the restandardized Minnesota Multiphasic Personality Inventory: MMPI-2. An administrative and interpretive guideline. Minneapolis (MN): University of Minnesota Press; 1989.
28. Heuchert JP, McNair DM. Profile of mood states. 2nd edition. Toronto: Multi-Health Systems; 2004.
29. Beck AT, Steer RA, Brown G. Beck depression inventory-II manual. San Antonio (TX): The Psychological Corporation; 1996.
30. Beck AT, Steer RA. Beck anxiety inventory manual. San Antonio (TX): The Psychological Corporation; 1987.
31. First MB, Spitzer RL, Gibbon M, et al. Structured clinical interview for DSM-IV axis I disorders (SCID-I), clinical version, user's guide. Arlington, VA: American Psychiatric Publishing; 1997.

Emerging Toxic Neuropathies and Myopathies

Hani A. Kushlaf, MB, BCh

KEYWORDS

- Toxic neuropathies • Toxic myopathies • Myopathy • Neuropathy
- Drug interactions

COMMENTARY ON EMERGING NEUROPATHIES AND MYOPATHIES FOR PSYCHIATRIC PRACTICE

Many medications cause a toxic myopathy or neuropathy. Toxic myopathies and/or neuropathies can occur as a direct or indirect adverse effect of medications. Several criteria should be met before the diagnosis of a toxic myopathy and/or neuropathy can be made. These include exposure to the drug before the onset of symptoms, the development of typical symptoms of toxicity known to be associated with the drug, and the resolution or improvement of symptoms with discontinuation of the offending drug in cases of direct toxicity. Increasing age, decreased clearance of medications by the liver or kidneys, and drug-drug interactions are factors that increase the likelihood of developing toxic myopathies and/or neuropathies. Genetic factors that predispose to toxic myopathies and/or neuropathies are identified in several instances (e.g., statin myopathy).

Psychiatrists in practice will encounter patients abusing alcohol and street drugs such as cocaine that can lead to toxic myopathies or neuropathies. Psychiatrists will also encounter patients with neuropsychiatric systemic lupus erythematosus who are treated with myotoxic medications (e.g., Hydroxychloroquine). Thus a well-rounded knowledge of toxic myopathies and neuropathies can be useful for the psychiatrist. The differential diagnosis of toxic myopathies and neuropathies is expanding rapidly and practical knowledge of these entities is becoming important.

This article originally appeared in the *August 2011 issue of Neurologic Clinics (Volume 29, Number 3)*.

The author has nothing to disclose.

Department of Neurology, University of Cincinnati, 260 Stetson Street, Suite 2300, PO Box 670525, Cincinnati, OH 45267-0525, USA

E-mail address: Hani.Kushlaf@uc.edu

KEY POINTS

- The mechanism by which medications cause myopathy or neuropathy is unknown in many instances (e.g. imatinib, and TNF-α antagonists).
- The presentation of statin myopathy is variable and range from relatively common myalgias to rare rhabdomyolysis.
- Measuring serum creatine kinase is important prior to starting statins.
- Hydroxychloroquine toxicity can culminate in respiratory failure.
- Vitamin E has been shown to reduce the incidence of cisplatin induced peripheral neuropathy.
- Although TNF-α antagonists are immunomodulators, they can cause different types of inflammatory neuropathies.
- Hypocupremia as a result of hyperzincemia typically causes myeloneuropathy, however, a motor neuron disorder-like syndrome develops in some patients.
- Autoimmune polyradiculoneuropathy can occur as a result of exposure to aerosolized porcine neural tissue.

MYOTOXINS
Statins

Statins are a group of drugs used to treat hypercholesterolemia. Approximately 30 million patients use statins in the United States,[1] with approximately 10% of them developing muscle-related complications that range from mild (myalgias) to serious (rhabdomyolysis). Predisposing factors to statin myotoxicity are shown in **Box 1**. Statins have been shown to be associated with several neuromuscular complications,[2] which are summarized in (**Box 2**).

In patients with statin myopathies, muscle biopsies often show nonspecific findings, such as cytochrome oxidase–negative fibers, increased fine lipid droplets, and ragged red fibers.[6]

Although myalgia is reported to develop in approximately 10% of patients taking statins, rhabdomyolysis remains a rare complication. Because diagnostic criteria do not exist for the definition of statin-associated myalgia, this condition is likely an underestimation of the true incidence.

The mechanism of statin-associated myopathy is largely unknown but is thought to be related to impaired prenylation (a process by which hydrophobic groups are added to proteins to facilitate cell membrane binding) of small proteins involved in signal transduction and altered protein glycosylation.[7]

Box 1
Risk factors for statin-induced myopathy

Atorvastatin>simvastatin, pravastatin, lovastatin>fluvastatin

Dual therapy with gemfibrozil and a statin

Underlying myopathy (muscular dystrophy, metabolic myopathy, inflammatory myopathy)

Genetic predisposition (eg, SLCO1B1)[3]

Drug-drug interactions (use of cytochrome P450 [CYP3A4] inhibitors, such as verapamil, itraconazole, cyclosporine)

Box 2
Neuromuscular complications described in patients on statins

Myalgia

Asymptomatic hyperCKemia

Acute rhabdomyolysis

Unmasking of other myopathies (eg, mitochondrial myopathy and other metabolic myopathies)

Immune-mediated myopathies

Myasthenia gravis (unmasking or aggravation)[4]

Rippling muscle disease[5]

Peripheral neuropathy

Patients with genetic mutations resulting in either muscular dystrophy or a metabolic myopathy are at a greater risk of developing a statin myopathy. Some patients with *LPIN1* mutation may develop severe myopathy after statin therapy.[8] Single nucleotide polymorphisms on *SLCO1B1*, which encodes the transporter associated with the hepatic uptake of all the statins except fluvastatin, are also associated with increased risk of statin-associated myopathies.[3]

Using statins safely requires regular monitoring for side effects. Specifically, creatine kinase (CK) levels should be measured in all patients before starting a statin. HyperCKemia at baseline suggests an underlying myopathy, and, in these patients, statin treatment has to be monitored cautiously or an alternative medication used. In patients who develop statin-induced myalgia, other causes for myalgias also have to be ruled out, which include fibromyalgia, hypothyroidism, and vitamin D deficiency. Of note, vitamin D deficiency has been shown to increase the risk of statin-induced myalgia.[9]

Asymptomatic hyperCKemia with CK levels less than 3 times normal should be monitored, and the statin drug can be continued. A rising CK level, myoglobinuria, or a CK level higher than ten times the normal level, should prompt immediate statin discontinuation. Discontinuing statin treatment should result in resolution of symptoms, CK normalization, and reversal of muscle biopsy changes within 2 to 3 months.

Patients taking statins can rarely develop an immune-mediated necrotizing myopathy.[10] These patients develop hyperCKemia and proximal muscle weakness, which continue to progress despite statin discontinuation. Although treatment with immunosuppressive agents (eg, steroids and methotrexate) may halt the progression, most patients suffer from some residual weakness.[10] After the statin is discontinued, one may alternatively use a bile acid sequestrant, such as colestipol, or a sterol absorption inhibitor, such as ezetimibe. Other options include using a statin that is less likely to cause a myopathy (eg, fluvastatin) or a statin with a longer half-life every 2 to 3 days instead of daily (eg, atorvastatin); Taking rosuvastatin every other day has been shown to increase its tolerability in patients who were rosuvastatin intolerant with everyday dosing while decreasing their low-density lipoprotein cholesterol levels to a desirable range.[11]

Pharmacogenetic screening does not seem to be cost effective at this point but may become available in the future. In patients with a severe hyperlipidemia who are in need of a fibrate, fenofibrate is a better choice than gemfibrozil because gemfibrozil is known to inhibit CYP2C8 and the hepatic organic anion transporter that are involved in hepatic uptake and metabolism of statins.[12]

Based on epidemiologic studies,[13,14] the incidence of developing a peripheral neuropathy while on a statin is low.

Imatinib Mesylate (Gleevec)

Imatinib is a tyrosine kinase inhibitor used to treat different types of cancer, including gastrointestinal stromal tumors and chronic myeloid leukemia.

In a 2008 case report, a 25-year-old patient receiving 400 mg of imatinib daily for treatment of desmoids tumors temporally developed CK elevations up to 1444 IU/L, with resolution of the hyperCKemia within days after discontinuing the medication.[15] On electromyography, a myopathic pattern was observed in the patient, with the authors concluding that imatinib could cause rhabdomyolysis.[15] After diagnosing rhabdomyolysis in a patient on imatinib, Gordon and colleagues[16] prospectively assessed the 1-year incidence of elevated CK levels in patients on imatinib. Of the 25 patients studied, they found hyperCKemia more than 2 times the upper limit of normal in 20 patients (80%) at some point during their treatment. This finding suggests that myopathy with imatinib may be common and may require routine screening in patients receiving therapy. On the contrary, rhabdomyolysis secondary to imatinib seems to be rare. The mechanism by which imatinib causes myopathy with hyperCKemia is unclear.

Daptomycin

Daptomycin is a lipopeptide antibiotic that works against gram-positive bacteria that has been shown to cause skeletal muscle toxicity in about 1.5% of patients.[17]

Kostrominova and colleagues[18] have shown that scattered muscle fibers are affected in early daptomycin toxicity. The mechanism of toxicity is postulated to be the result of daptomycin integration into the lipid rich outer leaflet of the sarcolemma with resultant calcium influx, which in turn leads to cell death. It is unclear if there is a predisposing factor to daptomycin myotoxicity.

Hydroxychloroquine

Hydroxychloroquine is an aminoquinoline antimalarial agent used for the treatment of connective tissue disorders such as rheumatoid arthritis and systemic lupus erythematosus. Hydroxychloroquine is known to cause mild to moderate vacuolar myopathy, and a recent report suggests that this condition can, at times, be severe and lead to respiratory failure.[19] Abdel-Hamid and colleagues[19] described 2 patients who developed this complication while on hydroxychloroquine. Discontinuing hydroxychloroquine did not improve their weakness. EMG showed positive sharp waves, myotonic discharges, and myopathic motor unit potentials. The CK level was normal in 1 patient and mildy elevated in the other patient. Muscle biopsy results showed fibers harboring rimmed vacuoles, atrophic fibers, and occasional necrotic and regenerating fibers. These rimmed vacuoles showed positive results for acid phosphatase and esterase. The autophagic vacuoles in the muscle biopsies are known features of hydroxychloroquine myotoxicity.

Highly Active Antiretroviral Therapy

Highly active antiretroviral therapy (HAART) is known to be associated with mitochondrial toxicity characterized by fatigue, lactic acidosis, and lipodystrophy.

Pfeffer and colleagues[20] reported on 3 patients who developed a chronic progressive ophthalmoplegia (CPEO) phenotype while on HAART. These patients have been on HAART for 15 to 18 years. One patient had an underlying mitochondrial DNA deletion, which was thought to be subclinical, and the patient expressed the CPEO phenotype after exposure to HAART. This patient had a levator palpebrae superioris biopsy during a procedure for ptosis that showed an abundance of ragged red fibers and cytochrome C oxidase (COX)-negative fibers. A quadriceps muscle biopsy in the same patient showed subsarcolemmal increases of oxidative enzyme activity and some COX-negative fibers. To further support the hypothesis of causation, the symptoms of one patient (fatigue, headache, and ptosis) improved after cessation of HAART.[20]

This report demonstrates that patients who present with a mitochondrial disease phenotype including CPEO, indeed, may have an underlying mitochondrial disease that became manifest with the use of mitochondrial toxic drugs.

NEUROMUSCULAR JUNCTION TOXINS
Tandutinib

Tandutinib (MLN 518, Millennium Pharmaceuticals, Cambridge, MA, USA) is a tyrosine kinase inhibitor currently in clinical trials for the treatment of glioblastoma multiforme. In one study[15] of 40 patients received a combination of tandutinib and bevacizumab, 6 developed muscle weakness. These patients developed facial weakness, neck weakness, and proximal greater than distal limb weakness. None of the patients developed ocular or pharyngeal weakness. Two patients had to discontinue the medication because of the weakness, even at a lower dose, whereas, 4 patients were able to tolerate the medication at lower doses. Repetitive nerve stimulation (RNS) showed a decremental response in patients evaluated with RNS, and, in 1 patient, improvement was shown after 1 week of drug discontinuation. Single-fiber EMG showed abnormal jitter with blocking in patients evaluated with single-fiber EMG.[21]

The mechanism of tandutinib neuromuscular junction toxicity is unclear, and studies are needed to clarify the pathophysiology underlying tandutinib toxic effect.

PERIPHERAL NERVE TOXINS
Bortezomib

Bortezomib (Velcade) is a selective 26S proteasome inhibitor used for the treatment of multiple myeloma and refractory or relapsed mantle cell lymphoma. Bortezomib is known to cause peripheral neuropathy that is mostly distal, sensory, and length dependent. In a study by Chaudhry and colleagues,[22] some patients developed a reversible demyelinating neuropathy and other patients developed perioral and scalp paresthesias, arguing for a sensory ganglionopathy as a possible site of toxicity. A single patient was reported to have an inflammatory neuropathy based on nerve biopsy findings and improvement on dexamethasone.[23] Cases of severe motor neuropathy have also been reported with bortezomib. In a cell culture study by Watanabe and colleagues,[24] the investigators demonstrated that compounds that induce heat shock protein 70 or lysosomal-associated membrane protein 2A are expected to improve or prevent bortezomib-induced peripheral neuropathy. Future clinical trials with the previously mentioned compounds are required to confirm and test this observation.

At present, the treatment is supportive with the treatment of neuropathic pain and use of orthoses. The sensory symptoms may improve as in the neuropathy caused by other chemotherapeutic agents.

Angel's Trumpet

Ingestion of angel's trumpet flowers (*Brugmansia suaveolens*; syn *Datura suaveolens*) is recently reported to cause the acute motor axonal neuropathy variant of Guillain-Barré syndrome.

In one case report, a 5-year-old boy developed a generalized weakness with difficulty in breathing, in addition to a left tonic pupil, after allegedly eating white flowers from the backyard.[25] Physical examination showed that the patient was generally weak, had generalized hyporeflexia, and had tachypnea (60 per minute). Magnetic resonance imaging (MRI) of the lumbar spine showed enhancement of the nerve roots of the cauda equina. Cerebrospinal fluid (CSF) analysis showed a cell count of 11, a protein level of 70 mg/dL, and a glucose level of 100 mg/dL. The patient did not respond to intravenous immunoglobulin (IVIG) and plasmaphresis. After recovery in 45 days, the patient reported eating white flowers from the backyard.

The mechanism by which angel trumpet causes Guillain-Barré is unclear; however, it could be related to an aberrant immune response similar to that seen after a variety of infections (Epstein-Barr virus, cytomegalovirus, hepatitis, varicella, and other herpes viruses, *Mycoplasma pneumoniae*, and *Campylobacter jejuni*), as well as immunizations that have been known to precede or to be associated with the illness. Angel's trumpet is in the nightshade family; it contains the alkaloids atropine, hyoscine, and scopolamine in a relatively high concentration, which makes it highly toxic. The predominant toxic syndrome seen in clinical practice is an anticholinergic syndrome. Unilateral tonic pupil has been reported in angel's trumpet intoxications.[26]

Because this is a single case report from a suspected ingestion, the association between angel's trumpet and the development of neuropathy is not clear at this time. It may be important to consider inquiring about plant ingestions in addition to tick paralysis when faced with a Guillain-Barré–like syndrome in a child.

Cisplatin

Cisplatin is a platinum-based antineoplastic alkylating agent used for the treatment of several cancers. It is well known that cisplatin causes chemotherapy-related peripheral neuropathy[27]; 90% of patients receiving a cumulative dose of 300 mg/m^2 or more develop a peripheral neuropathy. Recently, vitamin E was tried in a double-blind placebo-controlled trial to evaluate its neuroprotective effect.[28] A total of 108 patients receiving more than 300 mg/m^2 of cisplatin were randomized to vitamin E (400 mg/d) or placebo. The incidence of neurotoxicity was significantly lower in the vitamin E group (5.9%) compared with the placebo group (41.7%) ($P = .01$), demonstrating the potential effectiveness of vitamin E in preventing the neurotoxic effects of cisplatin.[28]

Oxaliplatin

Oxaliplatin is another platinum-based drug similar to cisplatin. Oxaliplatin causes a chronic sensory neurotoxicity similar to cisplatin, but it is also shown to cause acute motor nerve hyperexcitability that seems to be mechanistically different.[29] Hill and colleagues[30] demonstrated this phenomenon using motor nerve conduction studies and needle EMG. Repetitive compound motor action potentials were seen in 71% of patients. Abnormal high-frequency spontaneous motor fiber action potentials were seen in 100% of patients on days 2 to 4 after oxaliplatin treatment and decreased in frequency to 25% on days 14 to 20 after oxaliplatin treatment. The neuropathy induced by oxaliplatin seems to be long term and does not reverse completely on discontinuation.[31]

Tacrolimus

Tacrolimus is a potent immunosuppressant used to prevent organ transplant rejections (heart, kidney, and liver).

A recent case report showed that tacrolimus causes a toxic optic neuropathy. The frequency of this adverse effect seems to be rare.[32] The patient had undergone cardiac and renal transplants and developed asynchronous visual loss after taking tacrolimus for 5 years. MRI of the brain showed an optic nerve enlargement. Optic nerve biopsy showed evidence of demyelination without evidence of vasculitis. The patient did not improve after discontinuation of tacrolimus, which may indicate the irreversibility of this adverse effect. The investigators claimed that this report was the first report of toxic demyelination because most toxic agents cause axonopathies; however, it is unclear from the published report whether the demyelination is secondary to an axonal pathology and is clustered or primary, hence the need for teased fiber preparation to be done to differentiate between the two. The author argues that demyelination is secondary in this patient because the report showed endoneurial and perivascular macrophages in addition to axonal degeneration. The presence of these findings makes axonal degeneration the likely explanation of the observed demyelination.

Tumor Necrosis Factor α Antagonists

Tumor necrosis factor α (TNF-α) antagonists are important immunomodulators used for the treatment of several rheumatologic conditions, including rheumatoid arthritis, ankylosing spondylitis, psoriatic arthritis, Crohn disease, and ulcerative colitis. TNF-α antagonists include etanercept, infliximab, and adalimumab.

There are several reports associating the use of TNF-α antagonists with Guillain-Barré syndrome, Miller Fisher syndrome, chronic inflammatory demyelinating polyneuropathy, multifocal motor neuropathy with conduction block, mononeuropathy multiplex, and axonal sensorimotor polyneuropathies.[33]

Alshekhlee and colleagues[34] reported on 2 patients who developed chronic idiopathic demyelinating polyneuropathy while on treatment with etanercept and infliximab, respectively. The onset of symptoms varied between 2 weeks and 12 months of treatment with TNF-α antagonists. The mechanism of immune-mediated neuropathies in patients treated with TNF-α is unclear and remains to be fully explained. In contrast to previous reports, these 2 patients became dependent on immunosuppressive therapy instead of improvement on withdrawal of TNF-α antagonists.[34] Careful monitoring of patients is necessary to be aware of these immune-mediated neuropathies at an early stage during treatment with TNF-α antagonists.

Cobalt-Chromium

Ikeda and colleagues[35] reported on a patient who underwent a hip arthroplasty (cobalt-chromium prosthesis) 5 years before the development of symptoms. The symptoms consisted of gait disturbance, dysesthesias in all extremities, and auditory difficulties. The patient also had bilateral sensorineural hearing loss, which has been reported in patients with cobalt toxicity.[36]

Blood and sural nerve levels of cobalt and chromium were elevated and decreased after a revision surgery with ceramic-on-ceramic prosthesis; revision was also associated with improvement in symptoms. EMG showed absent sensory responses on nerve conduction studies. All motor responses were normal in nerve conduction studies. No needle examination was reported in the study.[35] A sural nerve biopsy showed decreased myelinated fiber density with a selective loss of large myelinated fibers. No significant inflammation was found. The findings on biopsy are in keeping with an axonal neuropathy. Sensory impairment in patients with artificial joints should raise a suspicion of this condition.

Zinc

Zinc is used in denture creams. Zinc induces intestinal metallothionein, which preferentially binds copper and is lost in feces with sloughed enterocytes. Hyperzincemia is shown in a study by Nations and colleagues[37] to be associated with hypocupremic myeloneuropathy. Myelopathy presents with spastic paraparesis, ataxia, and impairment of dorsal column sensations. The peripheral neuropathy tends to be sensory predominant and can be painful. Motor neuron disease–like presentation can occur in the setting of hypocupremia. Spinazzi and colleagues[38] questioned hyperzincemia as the sole cause of hypocupremia and pointed out that most patients with hypocupremic myeloneuropathy have other contributing factors, such as gastrointestinal surgeries, malnutrition, or malabsorption syndromes. A workup to exclude such factors is necessary in patients with hypocupremic myeloneuropathy. Discontinuing the use of zinc-based denture creams results in improvement of the hypocupremia and stabilization or mild improvement of the syndrome.

Ixabepilone

Ixabepilone is an epothilone B analogue that works as a microtubule stabilizer and is approved for use in the treatment of metastatic or locally advanced breast cancer (refractory or resistant). The most common adverse effects of ixabepilone are neutropenia and peripheral neuropathy.[39] The peripheral neuropathy is primarily sensory, is dose dependent, and reverses on discontinuation. The median time to improvement in symptoms is 4 to 6 weeks. Significant neuropathy usually develops after the third or fourth cycle of treatment. Depending on the severity of the neuropathy, lowering the dose may suffice in some patients.

Porcine Neural Tissue

Lachance and colleagues[40] reported on 24 patients who were exposed to aerosolized porcine neural tissue while working in 2 different swine abattoirs. A total of 21 patients developed an inflammatory painful sensory-predominant polyradiculoneuropathy with mild dysautonomia at the onset. The presentations included difficulty in walking, fatigue, sensory disturbances with burning, and aching pains. More than half the patients had an associated headache. Three patients developed aseptic meningitis, transverse myelitis, and meningoencephalitis, which were followed by a painful polyradiculoneuropathy. CSF analysis showed elevated CSF protein level in 18 of 21 tested patients and a pleocytosis in 3 of 21 tested patients. There was a preferential involvement of areas lacking in blood-brain barrier in all patients, such as dorsal root ganglia, dorsal roots, and distal sensory and motor nerves. The proximal involvement was identified on eliciting pain consistently with root stretching maneuvers, nerve conduction studies showing prolonged F-wave latencies and trigeminal blink responses, a thermoregulatory sweat testing showing a polyradicular pattern of sweat loss, and MRI showing enlargement and enhancement of nerve roots and ganglia. The involvement of distal sensory and motor nerves was identified on nerve conduction studies showing prolonged distal motor and sensory latencies, distal sweat loss on thermoregulatory sweat testing, and distal abnormalities on quantitative sensory testing. Sural nerve biopsies in 4 patients showed findings of inflammatory demyelination. Seventeen of the patients underwent treatment with immunosuppressive agents including intravenous methylprednisolone, IVIG, plasma exchange, and oral prednisone resulting in improvement in motor symptoms; however, most patients were left with residual pain and sensory symptoms. Autoimmunity developing after exposure to porcine neural tissue was suspected to be the cause of this syndrome.

SUMMARY

This article described new, and potentially new, toxic myopathies, neuropathies, and neuromuscular junction syndromes. Of the toxins discussed, there is little consensus as to the prevention or treatment of toxicity. In addition, the mechanism of toxicity or causation in many of the identified peripheral nerve toxins is still unclear. The identification of new toxic syndromes requires careful analysis of the clinical presentation of patients, in addition to paying close attention to demographic and occupational attributes. Further research is required to further elucidate the basic mechanisms underlying these toxic syndromes, thus identifying plans for prevention and treatment.

REFERENCES

1. Stagniti MN. Trends in statins utilization and expenditure for the U.S. civilian noninstitutionalized population, 2000 and 2005. Agency for Healthcare Research and Quality. Statistical brief #205, May 2008.
2. Mastalgia FL. Iatrogenic myopathies. Curr Opin Neurol 2010;23:445–9.
3. Link E, Parish S, Armitage J, et al. SLCO1B1 variants and statin-induced myopathy—a genome wide study. N Engl J Med 2008;359:789–99.
4. Purvin V, Kawasaki A, Smith KH, et al. Statin-associated myasthenia gravis: report of 4 cases and review of the literature. Medicine 2006;85:82–5.
5. Baker SK, Tarnopolsky MA. Sporadic rippling muscle disease unmasked by simvastatin. Muscle Nerve 2006;34:478–81.
6. Oskarsson B. Myopathy: five new things. Neurology 2011;76:S14.
7. Vaklavas C, Chatzizisis YS, Ziakas A, et al. Molecular basis of statin-associated myopathy. Atherosclerosis 2009;202:18–28.
8. Zeharia A, Shaag A, Houtkooper RH, et al. Mutations in LPIN1 cause recurrent acute myoglobinuria in childhood. Am J Hum Genet 2008;83:489–94.
9. Lee P, Greenfield JR, Campbell LV. Vitamin D insufficiency—a novel mechanism of statin-induced myalgia? Clin Endocrinol (Oxf) 2009;71:154–5.
10. Grable-Esposito P, Katzberg HD, Greenberg SA, et al. Immune-mediated necrotizing myopathy associated with statins. Muscle Nerve 2010;41:185–90.
11. Backes JM, Venero CV, Gibson CA, et al. Effectiveness and tolerability of every-other-day rosuvastatin dosing in patients with prior statin intolerance. Ann Pharmacother 2008;42:341–6.
12. Neuvonen PJ, Niemi M, Backman JT. Drug interactions with lipid-lowering drugs: mechanisms and clinical relevance. Clin Pharmacol Ther 2006;80:565–81.
13. Lovastatin Study Groups I Through IV. Lovastatin 5-year safety and efficacy study. Arch Intern Med 1993;153:1079–87.
14. Gaist D, Jeppesen U, Andersen M, et al. Statins and risk of polyneuropathy: a case-control study. Neurology 2002;58:1333–7.
15. Penel N, Blay JY, Adenis A. Imatinib as a possible cause of rhabdomyolysis. N Engl J Med 2008;358:2746–7.
16. Gordon JK, Magid SK, Makib RG, et al. Elevations of creatine kinase in patients treated with imatinib mesylate. Leuk Res 2010;34:827–9.
17. Rybak MJ. The efficacy and safety of daptomycin: first in a new class of antibiotics for Gram-positive bacteria. Clin Microbiol Infect 2006;12(Suppl 1):24–32.
18. Kostrominova TY, Hassett CA, Rader EP, et al. Characterization of skeletal muscle effects associated with daptomycin in rats. Muscle Nerve 2010;42:385–93.
19. Abdel-Hamid H, Oddis CV, Lacomis D. Severe hydroxychloroquine myopathy. Muscle Nerve 2008;38:1206–10.
20. Pfeffer G, Côté HC, Montaner JS, et al. Ophthalmoplegia and ptosis: mitochondrial toxicity in patients receiving HIV therapy. Neurology 2009;73:71–2.
21. Lehky TJ, Iwamoto FM, Kreisl TN, et al. Neuromuscular junction toxicity with tandutinib induces a myasthenic-like syndrome. Neurology 2011;76:236–41.

22. Chaudhry V, Cornblath DR, Polydefkis M, et al. Characteristics of bortezomib- and thalidomide-induced peripheral neuropathy. J Peripher Nerv Syst 2008;13: 275–82.

23. Saifee TA, Elliott KJ, Lunn MP, et al. Bortezomib-induced inflammatory neuropathy. J Peripher Nerv Syst 2010;15:366–8.

24. Watanabe T, Nagase K, Chosa M, et al. Schwann cell autophagy induced by SAHA, 17 AAG, or clonazepam can reduce bortezomib-induced peripheral neuropathy. Br J Cancer 2010;103:1580–7.

25. Sevketoglu E, Tatli B, Tuğcu B, et al. An unusual cause of fulminant Guillain-Barré syndrome: angel's trumpet. Pediatr Neurol 2010;43:368–70.

26. Andriol B, Povan A, Da Dolt L, et al. Unilateral mydriasis due to angel's trumpet. Clin Toxicol 2008;46:329–31.

27. Alberts DS, Noel JK. Cisplatin-associated neurotoxicity: can it be prevented? Anticancer Drugs 1995;6:369–83.

28. Pace A, Giannarelli D, Galiè E, et al. Vitamin E neuroprotection for cisplatin neuropathy: a randomized, placebo-controlled trial. Neurology 2010;74:762–6.

29. Lehky TJ, Leonard GD, Wilson RH, et al. Oxaliplatin-induced neurotoxicity: acute hyperexcitability and chronic neuropathy. Muscle Nerve 2004;29:387–92.

30. Hill A, Bergin P, Hanning F, et al. Detecting acute neurotoxicity during platinum chemotherapy by neurophysiological assessment of motor nerve Hyperexcitability. BMC Cancer 2010;10:451.

31. Park SB, Lin CS, Krishnan AV, et al. Long-term neuropathy after oxaliplatin treatment: challenging the dictum of reversibility. Oncologist 2011;16(5):708–16.

32. Venneti S, Moss HE, Levin MH, et al. Asymmetric bilateral demyelinating optic neuropathy from tacrolimus toxicity. J Neurol Sci 2011;301:112–5.

33. Stübgen JP. Tumor necrosis factor-alpha antagonists and neuropathy. Muscle Nerve 2008;37:281–92.

34. Alshekhlee A, Basiri K, Miles JD, et al. Chronic inflammatory demyelinating polyneuropathy associated with TNF-α antagonists. Muscle Nerve 2010;41:732–7.

35. Ikeda T, Takahashi K, Kabata T, et al. Polyneuropathy caused by cobalt-chromium metallosis after total hip replacement. Muscle Nerve 2010;42:140–3.

36. Oldenburg M, Wegner R, Baur X. Severe cobalt intoxication due to prosthesis wear in repeated total hip arthroplasty. J Arthroplasty 2009;24:825.e15–20.

37. Nations SP, Boyer PJ, Love LA, et al. Denture cream: an unusual source of excess zinc, leading to hypocupremia and neurologic disease. Neurology 2008;71: 639–43.

38. Spinazzi M, De Lazzari F, Tavolato B, et al. Myelo-opticoneuropathy in copper deficiency occurring after partial gastrectomy: do small bowel bacterial overgrowth syndrome and occult zinc ingestion tip the balance? J Neurol 2007;254: 1012–7.

39. Yardley DA. Proactive management of adverse events maintains the clinical benefit of ixabepilone. Oncologist 2009;14:448–55.

40. Lachance DH, Lennon VA, Pittock SJ, et al. An outbreak of neurological autoimmunity with polyradiculoneuropathy in workers exposed to aerosolized porcine neural tissue: a descriptive study. Lancet Neurol 2010;9:55–66.

Neurotoxic Emergencies

J. Dave Barry, MD[a,b,c],*, Brandon K. Wills, DO, MS[d,e,f]

KEYWORDS

- Poisoning • Emergency • Overdose • Neurology • Toxicology • Neurotoxins
- Seizures • Antidepressants

COMMENTARY ON NEUROTOXINS FOR PSYCHIATRIC PRACTICE

In this article, we highlight causative agents of neurotoxic emergencies, many of which are easily mistaken for acute psychiatric disorders. Understanding the wide variety of agents responsible for neurotoxic emergencies and the neurotransmitter interactions involved will help the psychiatrist identify and treat this challenging population.

The initial evaluation of a psychiatric patient hinges on identifying alternate causative medical, organic and toxic etiologies complicating the patient's presentation. The evaluation of psychiatric patients in the emergency environment is especially challenging due to the uncontrolled setting, uncertain history and the wide variety of potential organic and toxic etiologies that could be contributing to the patient's clinical presentation.

Medical treatment using pharmaceuticals includes a risk-benefit analysis, weighing anticipated benefit with the potential for harm. Acute or chronic toxicity from pharmaceuticals may manifest as an amplification of expected adverse drug reactions (ADR) or may have a distinct toxic syndrome. Treating clinicians primarily focus on beneficial and adverse effects of pharmaceuticals in therapeutic doses whereas medical toxicologists focus on toxicologic effects in acute or chronic overdose.

It is important to understand the side effect profile, ADRs, and drug-drug interactions for medications prescribed however, an understanding of how these xenobiotics manifest in overdose can also be useful for treating clinicians. Clinicians cannot predict or prevent intentional overdose, or control illicit drug use however; a reasonable

This article originally appeared in the *August 2011 issue of Neurologic Clinics (Volume 29, Number 3)*.

The views expressed in this article are those of the authors and do not reflect the official policy, position, or doctrine of the US Army, US Navy, DOD, or the US Government.

The authors have nothing to disclose.

[a] Emergency Medicine Residency Program, Naval Medical Center Portsmouth, Portsmouth, VA, USA; [b] Department of Emergency Medicine, Naval Medical Center Portsmouth, 620 John Paul Jones Circle, Portsmouth, VA 23708-2197, USA; [c] Uniformed Services University of the Health Sciences, Bethesda, MD, USA; [d] Virginia Commonwealth University Medical Center, Richmond, VA, USA; [e] Department of Emergency Medicine, Virginia Commonwealth University Health Center, Richmond, VA, USA; [f] Virginia Poison Center, PO Box 980522, Richmond, VA 23298, USA

* Corresponding author. 2605 Admiral Drive, Virginia Beach, VA 23451.

E-mail address: James.barry@med.navy.mil

http://dx.doi.org/10.1016/j.psc.2013.02.003
0193-953X/13/$ – see front matter © 2013 Elsevier Inc. All rights reserved.
psych.theclinics.com

risk-benefit analysis can be used when making treatment decisions recognizing that some pharmaceuticals are much more toxic in overdose than others.

We hope this article provides useful information to treating clinicians and furthers an understanding of acute care considerations for neurotoxic emergencies.

KEY POINTS

- Multiple xenobiotics producing acute excited mental status interact with the central biogenic amines, leading to a variety of toxic syndromes.
- Neurotoxic xenobiotics can alter GABA homeostasis, leading to acute depressed mental status in a variety of ways.
- Neuroleptic malignant syndrome is usually associated with rapid escalation of an antipsychotic or sudden discontinuation of anti-Parkinson medications. Symptoms develop over a period of 1 to 3 days, usually in sequential fashion, beginning with AMS and muscle rigidity.
- Cannabinoids have a linear dose-response relationship for inducing neuropsychiatric effects. At moderate doses, cannabinoids cause CNS depressant effects, including analgesia, euphoria, sedation, anxiolysis, and impairment of cognitive and psychomotor performance. Large doses can lead to adverse psychological effects primarily manifested by anxiety, panic attacks, agitation, acute psychosis, and paranoia.
- Acetylcholine antagonism produces the collection of symptoms commonly referred to as the anticholinergic syndrome: hyperthermia, tachycardia, flushed skin, anhydrosis, mydriasis, hypoactive bowel sounds, urinary retention, delirium, agitation, picking movements, hallucinations, and coma.

The symptoms and effects delineating a neurotoxic emergency vary depending on the viewpoint of the clinician. In general, agents causing acute life-threatening conditions have rapid mechanisms that severely disrupt major organ systems. This article focuses on agents causing rapid decompensation to a potentially life-threatening condition. The majority of these agents affect the central nervous system (CNS), thus the article is structured based on CNS effects: drug-induced and toxin-induced seizures, acute depressed mental status, and acute excited mental status. The final section highlights selected agents with primarily peripheral effects that meet the same criteria for an acute life-threatening condition.

A wide variety of poisons, toxins, drugs, chemicals, industrial agents, pesticides, and environmental agents have the potential to cause emergent neurotoxic effects. To avoid confusion, the authors use the term "xenobiotic" when discussing the various causative neurotoxic agents. A xenobiotic is a pharmacologically, endocrinologically, or toxicologically active substance not endogenously produced and therefore foreign to the organism.[1]

Neurotoxic xenobiotics produce symptoms in the victim through a wide array of different mechanisms, as shown in **Table 1**. Neurotoxic emergencies frequently affect the CNS through effects on neurotransmitters; therefore, much of this discussion focuses on the actions of specific neurotransmitters.

DRUG-INDUCED AND TOXIN-INDUCED SEIZURES

Seizures are a manifestation of many drug and toxin exposures or withdrawal syndromes. Some overdoses may include seizure amongst a myriad of other organ system toxicities, whereas others induce seizures as the primary manifestation of toxicity.

Table 1
Mechanisms of neurotoxic xenobiotics

Effect	Specific Mechanism
Cellular	Oxidative stress (free radicals, nucleophiles, or electrophiles)
	Alteration of membrane integrity
	Disruption of energy metabolism and/or regulation
	Altered regulation of gene expression
	Altered protein production
	Disruption of intracellular ion homeostasis
Metabolic	Stimulation or inhibition of enzymatic function
	Mimicking the actions of nutrients, hormones, or neurotransmitters
Neurotransmitter	Stimulation or blockade neurotransmitter receptors
	Altered release, uptake, and/or storage of neurotransmitters
	Altered neurotransmitter production or metabolism

Drug-induced and toxin-induced seizures (DTS) are typically generalized seizures, with status epilepticus occurring in approximately 4% to 10% of cases.[2,3] The epidemiology and incidence of DTS are not well known because seizures are not always tracked by regional poison centers. The California Poison Control Systems have provided the best view of agents most frequently implicated in DTS through a series of investigations over the last 17 years.[2–4] Over this time period, the proportion of DTS from tricyclic antidepressants (TCA), stimulants, and theophylline fell while anticholinergic antihistamines and isoniazid remained fairly constant. Their most recent prospective series of DTS found antidepressants were most common (33%) followed by stimulants (15%), antiepileptics (12%), and anticholinergic antihistamines (10%).[2] Of note, citalopram and escitalopram were absent from their 1994 and 2003 series yet comprised 8% of cases in the most recent review.[2] A comprehensive review of toxin-related seizures was recently published.[5] This section discusses some of the more common and newer pharmaceuticals implicated in DTS.

Psychiatric Agents

Tricyclic antidepressants
TCAs have multiple pharmacologic effects including serotonin and norepinephrine reuptake inhibition, central and peripheral anticholinergic and antihistamine effects, peripheral α_1 antagonism, and fast sodium channel blockade.[6] A recent series documenting prevalence of clinical outcomes in amitriptyline overdose reported seizures in 6%, hypotension in 10%, coma in 29%, and wide QRS complex or ventricular dysrhythmia in 30%.[7] Acidemia from seizures or hypotension can decrease TCA protein binding, resulting in worsening toxicity.[8] Seizures are treated primarily with benzodiazepines. Boluses of sodium bicarbonate are useful for the cardiovascular effects of TCA poisoning by providing a sodium bolus as well as raising the serum pH.[6,8]

Bupropion
Bupropion is a mixed dopamine and norepinephrine reuptake inhibitor, well known to lower the seizure threshold in therapeutic doses and induce seizures in overdose.[9] Of all drug-induced seizures reported to a regional poison center, 14.9% were due to bupropion.[2] Another poison center review of bupropion overdoses reported generalized seizures in 32% of cases, 32% of which occurred more than 8 hours after overdose.[10] In this series, 19% of patients who seized also exhibited hallucinations. One patient did not manifest their first seizure until 24 hours after ingestion.

Citalopram

Citalopram overdose is frequently associated with QTc prolongation and seizures.[11] One 7-year review found seizures in 8% of citalopram overdoses; however, nearly half of the cases involved coingestants.[12] Escitalopram is the S-enantiomer of citalopram and produces substantially fewer seizures in overdose.[13,14]

Antiepileptic drugs

Seizures can paradoxically occur from overdose of anticonvulsants. This phenomenon is unlikely to occur in γ-aminobutyric acid (GABA)-mediated anticonvulsants but is seen in anticonvulsants with mixed receptor effects. Traditional anticonvulsants known to cause seizures in overdose are carbamazepine and, to a lesser extent, phenytoin.[15–17] The authors have less clinical experience with newer anticonvulsants, but seizures appear to occur frequently in overdose. Lamotrigine has been associated with seizures and nonconvulsive status epilepticus in both therapeutic dosing[18–20] and overdose.[21,22] Topirimate[23,24] and tiagabine[25–27] have also been reported to cause seizures in overdose.

Drugs of Abuse

Acute intoxication or drug withdrawal from several different classes can result in seizures. The stimulant class includes a diverse range of illicit drugs including amphetamines (illicit and medicinal), designer amphetamines, cocaine, and methylxanthines. Manifestations of stimulant overdose include a sympathomimetic toxidrome manifested by tachycardia, hypertension, mydriasis, diaphoresis, agitation, and tremor. Generalized seizures are frequently seen in moderate to severe cases.[28–30] Methylxanthine overdose can manifest with significant tachycardia, hypotension rather than hypertension, dysrhythmias, and refractory seizures.[29] Animal models and human series suggest hyperthermia in the setting of stimulant overdose is a surrogate of severe poisoning and increased mortality.[31–34]

The sympathomimetic toxidrome is frequently seen in moderate to severe sedative-hypnotic withdrawal. Seizures from drug withdrawal are observed primarily with ethanol,[35] sedative-hypnotics (eg, benzodiazepines, barbiturates), and baclofen.[36–38] It is uncommon for opioid withdrawal to cause seizures except in neonates born to opioid-dependent mothers.[39]

Opioids

The vast majority of opioids do not cause seizures in acute overdose or in withdrawal. A few notable exceptions are discussed here.

Tramadol

Tramadol is a synthetic analgesic with weak μ-receptor effects as well as serotonin and norepinephrine reuptake inhibition.[40] Case series of tramadol overdoses documented generalized seizures in 8% to 54% of cases, 45% to 63% being single seizures.[41–43] Other complications include rhabdomyolysis, acute kidney injury, and serotonin toxicity.[44,45]

Propoxyphene

Overdose of propoxyphene in some ways can mimic tricyclic antidepressant overdose with CNS depression, wide-complex dysrhythmias due to fast sodium channel blockade, and seizures.[46–48] In November 2010, propoxyphene was removed from United States markets, and removal has been under way since 2009 across Europe.

Meperidine

Meperidine, a synthetic opioid, is demethylated to the neurotoxic metabolite normeperidine.[49] Patients with renal insufficiency or receiving continuous infusions through patient-controlled analgesia devices are at particular risk for neurotoxicity and seizures.[50]

Other Agents

Isoniazid

Isoniazid (INH), a hydrazine used for tuberculosis, is well known for causing refractory seizures in overdose. Hydrazines can also be found in some types of rocket fuel and in the toxic mushroom *Gyromitra esculenta*. Hydrazines inhibit pyridoxine phosphokinase resulting in a functional vitamin B6 deficiency, an essential cofactor for GABA synthesis. INH overdose may include the triad of coma, severe lactic acidosis, and refractory seizures.[51]

Treatment

Decontamination considerations

Gastrointestinal decontamination options include gastric lavage, activated charcoal, and whole bowel irrigation. Gastric lavage is generally not recommended for most overdoses.[52] Single-dose activated charcoal is theoretically effective for most organic substances except for metals, hydrocarbons, alcohols, and caustics. Its efficacy for preventing absorption drops off sharply by 2 to 3 hours post ingestion.[53] Activated charcoal is contraindicated for patients with CNS depression, significant delirium, high risk for seizures, or an unprotected airway due to risks of pulmonary aspiration.[53] Whole bowel irrigation (WBI) involves the administration of polyethylene glycol solution at a rate of 1 to 2 liters per hour until the rectal effluent is clear. Although WBI has theoretical advantages for substances not absorbed by activated charcoal and sustained-release products, its routine use is not currently recommended.[54] It is also difficult to achieve complete bowel decontamination.[55] As mentioned with activated charcoal, neurotoxic overdoses resulting in alteration of consciousness and seizures increase the risk of pulmonary aspiration.

Enhanced elimination considerations

Enhancing the elimination of drugs or toxins can be accomplished through multidose activated charcoal (MDAC), urinary alkalinization, and hemodialysis. Drug overdoses likely to cause seizures that are amenable to MDAC include theophylline, carbamazepine, and quinine.[56] As with single-dose activated charcoal, patients with seizures or unprotected airway represent a significant risk for aspiration. Urinary alkalinization involves the administration of bicarbonate to raise urine pH above 7.5. It is useful to enhance the elimination of salicylates in moderate to severe poisonings.[57] Hemodialysis is also useful for moderate to severe toxicity from salicylates, lithium, and theophylline overdoses.[58]

Focused treatment

Initial management of the seizing patient includes attention to the airway, breathing, and circulation; establishing peripheral intravenous access, starting supplemental oxygen, bedside glucose determination, giving empiric anticonvulsant therapy, and treating other underlying sequelae due to overdose (eg, rhabdomyolysis or hyperthermia). Consultation with a medical toxicologist is useful for providing guidance on decontamination, enhanced elimination, resuscitative interventions, and antidotes.

DTS, which are frequently short lived and self limited, may not require anticonvulsant therapy. However, approximately 4% to 10% of DTS result in status epilepticus.[2,3]

Evidence-based approaches to treating drugs and DTS are lacking. Recommendations are frequently extrapolated from epilepsy research, pharmacologic mechanisms, and anecdotal experience. For most cases of DTS, anticonvulsant treatment should be focused on GABA agonists. Benzodiazepines remain first-line therapy for DTS. Lorazepam or diazepam are generally preferred, but barbiturates can also be used. Unlike seizures from drug overdose, severe delirium tremens may require massive doses of benzodiazepines to achieve control.[59,60] Propofol is an intravenous anesthetic that has been effective in controlling severe delirium tremens refractory to other agents.[61,62] It may be tried as a second-line therapy for refractory DTS.[63,64]

Phenytoin should not be considered first-line or second-line therapy for DTS. Phenytoin is not expected to be effective for the majority of DTS, and may exacerbate seizures with cocaine, lidocaine, theophylline, and organochlorine insecticides.[65] There is little evidence regarding the efficacy of valproic acid or levetiracetam for DTS, but because they have been used for non-DTS status epilepticus, are well tolerated, available as an intravenous bolus, and are GABA agonists, they would be reasonable to try as a third-line therapy.[66] One murine model evaluated 13 anticonvulsants' ability to prevent seizures induced by bupropion.[67] The investigators determined that carbamazepine, lamotrigine, phenytoin, and tiagabine were not effective at attenuating seizures.

Pyridoxine is indicated for isoniazid overdose with either seizure or coma.[68] It is given as an empiric dose of 5 g or at a dose equivalent to the amount of INH ingested if this is known.[69]

ACUTE DEPRESSED MENTAL STATUS

Chemical balance within the CNS is principally maintained by GABA as the predominant inhibitory neurotransmitter and by glutamate, the predominant excitatory neurotransmitter.[70] A wide variety of other neurotransmitters, ion channels, and modulators contribute in a less significant way to this balance, and are less understood. Stimulation by GABA, γ-hydroxybutyrate (GHB), opioids, and cannabinoids all have the potential to produce acute depressed mental status.

γ-Aminobutyric Acid

There are 3 distinct GABA receptor subtypes: $GABA_A$, $GABA_B$, and $GABA_C$. $GABA_A$ receptors are ligand-gated chloride ion channels. In addition to the GABA binding sites, there are others where multiple xenobiotics and endogenous modulators can bind, altering the chloride current. Xenobiotics causing acute depressed mental status commonly target this $GABA_A$ receptor complex. $GABA_B$ are G-protein–coupled receptors that ultimately alter calcium or potassium currents.[71] $GABA_C$ are ligand-gated chloride ion channels that are structurally, functionally, and pharmacologically distinct from $GABA_A$.[72] The clinical importance of $GABA_C$ receptors is poorly understood.

Neurotoxic xenobiotics can alter GABA homeostasis, leading to acute depressed mental status in a variety of ways. The most common mechanism is through indirect stimulation of $GABA_A$ receptors, increasing the affinity of GABA for its receptor, or increasing the frequency or duration of chloride channel opening. Both benzodiazepine and barbiturate classes of drugs,[73–76] steroids,[76] various anesthetics,[76] and other xenobiotics exert their clinical effects through these mechanisms. Muscimol, a direct $GABA_A$ agonist, is found naturally in *Aminita muscaria* (fly agaric) and *Aminita pantherina* (panther cap) mushrooms, along with ibotenic acid, an excitatory glutamic acid receptor agonist.[77] Baclofen is a direct $GABA_B$ receptor agonist. Commonly administered via an intrathecal pump, baclofen overdose can cause profound CNS depression.[78]

GABA concentrations in the brain can be increased by stimulating GABA production, regulated by the enzyme glutamic acid decarboxylase (GAD) or by decreasing GABA metabolism, regulated by GABA transaminase. These mechanisms contribute at least partially to the clinical effects of sodium valproate,[79,80] gabapentin,[81] and vigabatrin.[82] Tiagabine similarly increases GABA concentrations by inhibiting GABA reuptake through blockade of the GABA transporter, GAT-1.[83]

Treatment of acute depressed mental status caused by GABA stimulation is primarily supportive, with specific attention to the patient's protective airway reflexes, and ventilatory and oxygenation status. Flumazenil binds to the benzodiazepine site on the GABA receptor, competitively inhibiting benzodiazepines and related xenobiotics. Although flumazenil effectively reverses the CNS effects of these agents,[84] it is not recommended for routine use on all altered or comatose patients because of the potential for inducing withdrawal in the chronic user, provoking seizures in both epileptic and nonepileptic patients, and unmasking excitatory coingestants. Reasonable use of flumazenil would be in benzodiazepine overdose in naïve patients and iatrogenic benzodiazepine overdose from procedural sedation.[85]

γ-Hydroxybutyrate

GHB is an endogenous neurotransmitter. Marketed as sodium oxybate, a pharmaceutical treatment for narcolepsy, it is also a popular drug of abuse. GHB is both a precursor and a metabolite of GABA. Structurally similar, these compounds share a common catabolic and metabolic pathway. GHB precursors are widely used in industry, but are also commonly abused recreationally as food supplements, and are rarely implicated as incapacitating agents (facilitating sexual assault).[86]

Although similar to GABA, GHB has its own distinct G-protein–linked receptor. The mechanisms of action of GHB are incompletely understood. Whether through interactions at the GHB receptor or by neuromodulation at other receptors, GHB alters CNS concentrations of GABA, dopamine, serotonin, norepinephrine, opioids, and glutamate.[87,88]

Physiologic concentrations of GHB interact primarily at the GHB receptors.[88] The administration of exogenous GHB, either for therapeutic or recreational reasons, dramatically increases CNS concentrations. The effects of supraphysiologic GHB concentrations are primarily mediated at $GABA_B$ receptors, but additional less well described interactions probably also occur.[87–89]

Supraphysiologic GHB concentrations produce varying degrees of CNS depression ranging from disinhibition (agitated delirium), to mild (sedation, ataxia, dizziness), to severe (coma, respiratory depression, apnea, death).[90–92] Other common symptoms include bradycardia, hypothermia, and vomiting. Myoclonus and convulsive activity has been reported with GHB toxicity, but it is unclear whether these are true seizures.[90,93] Abrupt awakening from deep coma is commonly reported in association with GHB toxicity.[94] With chronic use, a withdrawal syndrome, clinically similar to sedative-hypnotic withdrawal, can manifest after abrupt discontinuation.

Treatment of GHB toxicity is primarily symptomatic and supportive. Various agents (flumazenil, naloxone, physostigmine) have been suggested as antidotes for GHB toxicity, but none have shown consistent efficacy. GHB withdrawal is treated in a similar fashion to sedative-hypnotic withdrawal, with high-dose benzodiazepine as the first-line agent. Refractory GHB withdrawal has been described. These cases can be controlled with cross-tolerant sedative-hypnotics such as benzodiazepines, barbiturates, chloral hydrate, or propofol.[95,96] Baclofen has also been suggested as a treatment for GHB withdrawal.[97]

Opioids

Opioid receptors are distributed widely throughout the CNS, spinal cord, and peripheral nervous system (PNS). Although extensively studied, the clinical effects mediated by their G-protein–mediated receptors are not completely understood. The classic Greek nomenclature (μ, κ, δ) used to describe opioid receptors is transitioning to one recommended by the International Union on Receptor Nomenclature (MOP/OP_3, KOP/OP_2, DOP/OP_1). There are 3 primary opioid receptors, each with their own specific subtypes, and a few less well described minor receptors. Each receptor type is distributed differently throughout the human body and imparts different clinical effects.

The μ (mu) opioid receptor (MOP, OP_3) was the first to be described as the morphine-binding site and is probably the best understood. Although there are 2 distinct subtypes (μ_1/OP_{3A}, μ_2/OP_{3B}), there are no known selective subtype xenobiotics. μ receptors mediate most of the clinical effects commonly attributed to opioids: analgesia, euphoria, sedation, respiratory depression, decreased gastrointestinal motility, and physical dependence.[98] κ (kappa) opioid receptors (KOP, OP_2) are concentrated in the spinal cord, mediating primarily spinal analgesia, miosis, and dysphoria. δ (delta) receptors (DOP, OP_1) are less well understood but may contribute to the psychomimetic and dysphoric properties of opioids. A fourth nonclassic opioid receptor, the nociceptin/orphanin FQ receptor (NOP, OP_4), was defined using DNA sequencing, but a clinical role has not yet been described.[98,99]

Pure opioid agonists frequently produce acute depressed mental status in conjunction with the classic opioid toxic syndrome: CNS depression, respiratory depression, and miosis.[100] Some opioid xenobiotics possess additional mechanisms of action (meperidine, tramadol, propoxyphene, dextromethorphan), thus the toxic presentation may include symptoms not classic for opioids and/or lack some symptoms of the classic opioid toxidrome.

Treatment of opioid toxicity focuses on early support of ventilation and oxygenation in addition to symptomatic care. Gastrointestinal decontamination should be considered based on the clinical situation. Opioid antagonists competitively inhibit the binding of opioid agonists to opioid receptors. Having a higher affinity for opioid receptors than opioid xenobiotics, they reverse the clinical effects of most opioid agonists.[98,101] Naloxone is the most commonly used opioid antagonist. The goal of opioid antagonist therapy is to restore adequate spontaneous ventilation and ensure that protective airway reflexes remain intact, while avoiding precipitation of acute withdrawal. Thus, the lowest possible dose that allows for adequate oxygenation and airway protection should be used.

Cannabinoids

Tetrahydrocannabinol (Δ^9-THC), cannabidiol (CBD), and cannabinol (CBN) are the most prevalent natural cannabinoids or phytocannabinoids, with the most potent being Δ^9-THC. Although categorized as a CNS depressant, it is extremely uncommon for cannabinoid toxicity to cause acute depressed mental status significant enough to be considered a neurotoxic emergency. Over the last few years, however, there has been resurgence in interest in cannabinoids due to the popularity of synthetic cannabinoid use.

Synthetic cannabinoids have become a popular "legal high," usually in the form of herbal blends purportedly sprayed with potent synthetic cannabinoids. Initially the most common herbal blends were sold under the brand name "spice." Recently, this term seems to have become short-hand for a variety of similar products containing synthetic cannabinoids (Genie, K2, Spice Diamond, Spice Gold, Spice Silver,

Yucatan Fire, Zohai, and so forth).[102] These products are marketed as incense blends, avoiding regulatory drug control.[102,103] Synthetic cannabinoids are reported to be more potent than their phytocannabinoid cousins.[102] Attributing the symptoms and complications of "spice" use to synthetic cannabinoids is difficult, due to the different combinations of additives used in these products.

Two distinct cannabinoid receptors have been characterized (CB1, CB2), both of which are G-protein–mediated receptors (GPMR). Globally, CB1 receptors are localized primarily in the brain, spinal cord, and testis, where the CB2 receptors are localized peripherally in immune tissues: leukocytes, splenocytes, and microglia.[104–106] Within the CNS, the cannabinoid system is thought to act as a negative feedback mechanism to dampen synaptic release of both excitatory and inhibitory neurotransmitters including glutamate, GABA, noradrenaline, dopamine, serotonin (5-HT), acetylcholine, and opioids.[106–108] Cannabinoid receptors are the most prevalent GPMR in the brain, with the highest concentrations in the basal ganglia and cerebellum.[106,108]

Cannabinoids have a linear dose-response relationship for inducing neuropsychiatric effects,[107,109,110] which can result in a higher propensity for adverse effects using potent synthetic cannabinoids. At moderate doses, cannabinoids cause CNS depressant effects, including analgesia, euphoria, sedation, anxiolysis, and impairment of cognitive and psychomotor performance.[107–109] Although clinically significant acute toxicity is uncommon, large doses of cannabinoids can lead to adverse psychological effects primarily manifested by anxiety, panic attacks, agitation, acute psychosis, and paranoia.[107,109,111] Peripheral effects include dry mouth, palpitations, tachycardia, and postural hypotension.[109]

Tolerance to the effects of cannabinoids is fairly well described.[107,108] Although psychiatric illness is associated with chronic cannabis use, there is no evidence that this relationship is causal.[106,108] A mild withdrawal syndrome has been demonstrated after cessation of heavy cannabinoid use manifested by the following: cravings, anorexia, insomnia, weight loss, irritability, restlessness, and autonomic effects.[107,108,110,112]

ACUTE EXCITED MENTAL STATUS

Although glutamic acid is the predominant excitatory neurotransmitter in the CNS, its interactions with xenobiotics are less well understood than those of the central biogenic amines. Multiple xenobiotics producing acute excited mental status interact with the central biogenic amines, leading to a variety of toxic syndromes discussed here. The complex and incompletely understood interactions of glutamic acid are then addressed.

Central Biogenic Amines

There are 5 biogenic amine neurotransmitters: histamine, 5-HT, and the 3 catecholamines dopamine (DA), norepinephrine (NE), and epinephrine (EPI). All 5 share common and incompletely understood interactions within the CNS. EPI and histamine have less predominant interactions, ultimately mediating CNS-excited mental status, so they are not discussed in this section.

NE, DA, and 5-HT share similar synthesis, storage, and degradation pathways within the CNS. DA is produced from tyrosine intracellularly in a 2-step enzymatic process involving tyrosine hydroxylase and amino acid decarboxylase. 5-HT utilizes a parallel process, with tryptamine instead of tyrosine as the parent compound. DA β-hydroxylase converts DA to NE after packaging into the nerve-ending vesicles. All 3 are removed from the synapse into the nerve ending by specific reuptake transporters. Although these transporters have high affinity for their parent compounds, they are also somewhat nonspecific, facilitating the transport of similarly structured amines and xenobiotics as well. After reuptake into the synapse, degradation of NE, DA, and 5-HT is primarily performed by monoamine oxidase (MAO).

Receptors for NE, DA, and 5-HT are widely distributed throughout the body. At least 9 different subtypes of NE receptor have been identified,[113] but only α_2 adrenergic receptors play a dominant central role. There are 5 distinct but closely related G-protein–coupled DA receptors, all with broad expression patterns peripherally and centrally.[114] Similarly, 5-HT has 7 major classes of receptor and multiple subtypes.[71] With the exception of 5-HT$_3$ receptors, which are ligand-gated ion channels, all 5-HT receptors are coupled to G proteins.[115]

Amphetamines

Amphetamines and the diverse group of phenethylamine analogues exert their effects indirectly by stimulating NE, DA, and/or 5-HT release, by blocking the reuptake of neurotransmitter into the neuron, and by inhibiting MAO.[116,117] Modifications of the amphetamine structure influence which neurotransmitter is predominantly affected. Amphetamine analogues with prominent serotonergic activity, such as 3,4-methylenedioxymethamphetamine (MDMA, "ecstasy"), yield more intense hallucinogenic properties. Mescaline, the active alkaloid in peyote (*Lophophora williamsii*), shares similar serotonergic effects.[118]

Recently, the synthetic amphetamine analogues mephedrone and methylenedioxypyrovalerone (MDPV) have been found in products sold as "novelty bath salts" ("ivory wave", "vanilla sky", and so forth) on Web sites and in specialty stores.[119] These products share structural similarity with cathinone, the active ingredient in the *Catha edulis* plant (Khat). Metcathinone ("cat", "jeff") is also a synthetic analogue of cathinone.[120]

Cocaine

Similar to amphetamines, cocaine exerts its effects by blocking the reuptake of biogenic amines and thus increasing levels in the nerve terminal.[100,121] Cocaine also increases the concentration of excitatory amino acids,[122] possibly contributing to its clinical effects. Unlike amphetamines, cocaine also possess sodium channel blocking effects (Class I antiarrhythmic) similar to cyclic antidepressants, increasing the risk for cardiac dysrhythmias.[30,121]

Indolealkylamines

Indolealkylamines, or tryptamines, share structural similarity with 5-HT, making this class potent hallucinogens. Psilocybin-containing mushrooms ("magic mushrooms"), 5-methoxy-*N,N*-diisopropyltryptamine ("Foxy", "Foxy methoxy"), *N,N*-dimethyltryptamine (DMT, Ayahuasca, "Businessman's Lunch"), and α-methyltryptamine (AMT, "spirals") all share similar properties due to their common tryptamine-like structure. Lysergic acid diethylamide (LSD) and its analogues, like those found in morning glory seeds (*Ipomea violacea*), also share structural similarities to 5-HT.[100]

Treatment considerations

Treatment of acute excited mental status due to biogenic amines is symptom and side-effect directed. Hyperthermia should be aggressively treated with active cooling and aggressive control of agitation. Benzodiazepines are first-line agents for agitation and signs of peripheral sympathetic stimulation (tachycardia, hypertension, tachypnea). Alternative GABA agonists (short-acting barbiturates, propofol) can be used for intractable agitation. Persistent hypertension should be controlled with phentolamine or nitrates (nitroglycerine, nitroprusside). Although controversial, β-adrenergic blockers are relatively contraindicated as the resultant unopposed α-adrenergic effects may worsen coronary vasospasm and end-organ toxicity.[123–125] Wide-complex tachydysrhythmias should be treated with sodium bicarbonate. Gastrointestinal decontamination with activated charcoal could be considered for early ingestions. Contraindications are similar to those discussed for seizures. Finally, diligence in watching for and preventing other complications, including rhabdomyolysis, subarachnoid or intraparenchymal hemorrhage, myocardial ischemia, ischemic bowel, and other end-organ effects, is warranted.

Neuroleptic Malignant Syndrome

Neuroleptic malignant syndrome (NMS) is a relatively rare, but potentially fatal complication of treatment with antipsychotic drugs characterized by altered mental status (AMS) (ranging from lethargy, agitation, stupor, to coma), muscle rigidity (classically described as "lead pipe" rigidity[126–128]), fever, and autonomic dysfunction (including tachycardia, tachypnea, hypertension or hypotension, diaphoresis, and possibly cardiac arrhythmias). NMS is usually associated with rapid escalation of an antipsychotic or sudden discontinuation of antiparkinson medications. Neuromuscular manifestations are due to decreased dopaminergic neurotransmission or DA_2 blockade in various CNS locations.[128–130] Symptoms develop over a period of 1 to 3 days, usually in a sequential fashion, beginning with AMS and muscle rigidity.[130]

Initial treatment focuses on early recognition and prompt withdrawal of any dopamine antagonists along with aggressive supportive care, benzodiazepines, and active cooling measures. Dopamine agonists (bromocriptine or amantadine) and dantrolene sodium (based on its efficacy in malignant hyperthermia) have been used anecdotally with varying benefits, but neither has been shown to be consistently superior to supportive care alone.[129–131] Nondepolarizing neuromuscular blockade and mechanical ventilation may be necessary to control rigidity and hyperthermia in severe cases. Electroconvulsive therapy has been performed in patients exhibiting resistant symptoms with anecdotal improvement.[127,129,130] NMS should be considered a diagnosis of exclusion and requires a thorough investigation for alternative causes of AMS, fever, and/or muscle rigidity.

Serotonin Toxicity

Serotonin toxicity is a similar syndrome, characterized by AMS (confusion, agitation, anxiety, hallucinations, lethargy, coma), autonomic instability (flushing, shivering, hypertension, hyperthermia, tachycardia, tachypnea), and neuromuscular abnormalities (tremor, hyperreflexia, myoclonus, muscular rigidity).[132] The manifestations of serotonin toxicity can vary across a spectrum of severity, with the most extreme resembling NMS. Hyperreflexia and clonus in serotonin toxicity are characteristic, being noticeably greater in the lower extremities than in the upper extremities.[126] Unlike NMS, the symptoms occur rapidly, within hours after the initiation of a serotonergic agent, and can escalate quickly to a life-threatening condition.[126,133] The syndrome is thought to be due to increases in extracellular concentrations of serotonin with subsequent stimulation of $5\text{-}HT_{2A}$ and other serotonin and monoaminergic receptors.[126,132–134] Although several diagnostic criteria have been proposed,[133,135] these investigators recommend against using them in clinical practice because it could cause oversight and thus delay treatment of atypical cases. Instead, a low threshold should be maintained for diagnosing serotonin toxicity in any patient taking serotonergic xenobiotics that develops a combination of AMS, autonomic findings, and neuromuscular abnormality. Treatment intensity can be tailored to symptom severity but should include discontinuation any serotonergic agents and supportive care.

Supportive measures include benzodiazepines for autonomic overactivity and active cooling for hyperthermia. Vasoactive medications, nondepolarizing neuromuscular blockade, and mechanical ventilation may be necessary in severe cases. 5-HT$_{2A}$ antagonists (cyproheptadine, chlorpromazine) have been suggested as adjuncts in moderate to severe cases, but their benefit in humans is largely anectdotal.[126,133]

Glutamic Acid

As mentioned previously, glutamic acid is the predominant excitatory neurotransmitter in the CNS. Glutamic acid is the immediate precursor to GABA, the predominant inhibitory CNS neurotransmitter. Glutamate is closely regulated by the brain, which dedicates up to two-thirds of its energy metabolism to control the reuptake and recycling of this neurotransmitter.[136] There are 11 different types of glutamate receptor: 8 are G-protein mediated (metabotropic), the other 3 being ligand-gated ion channels (ionotropic). The ionotropic receptors are named after the agonist used to identify them. Of these, the N-methyl-D-aspartic acid (NMDA) receptor is the most thoroughly studied. A unique aspect of the NMDA receptor is that it is gated both by ligands and by voltage.[137,138] Magnesium binds to a site within the ion channel, blocking the flow of calcium across the neuronal membrane.[136] In addition to glutamate binding sites, the NMDA channel also has sites for the inhibitory neurotransmitter glycine.[137] The glycine site, similar to the indirect stimulation of GABA receptors, alters the affinity of NMDA for glutamate and varies the frequency or duration of channel opening, but does not, by itself, induce channel opening.[136]

Phencyclidine, Ketamine, Dextromethorphan

Phencyclidine (PCP), ketamine, and dextromethorphan (DXM) bind to an independent site (the PCP binding site)[139] on the NMDA receptor, inhibiting ionic flow. The clinical effects of this inhibition is a "dissociative effect," causing a dissociation between the thalamoneocortical and limbic systems, and preventing the higher centers from perceiving visual, auditory, or painful stimuli.[140] Muscle tone is maintained; therefore, airway protective measures are preserved. In addition to profound anesthetic and analgesic effects, mild cardiovascular stimulation (tachycardia, hypertension, diaphoresis),[140,141] and horizontal, vertical, or rotatory nystagmus[142] are frequently seen. Anxiety, agitation, combativeness, coma, neuromuscular rigidity, and seizures are associated with high doses and/or coingestion of other neuroactive xenobiotics. Hallucinations and nightmares can be seen as subjects emerge from their dissociation; an effect coined as the "emergence phenomenon."[140,142] Treatment is essentially supportive, with benzodiazepine sedation if necessary. The development or coexistence of complications, such as rhabdomyolysis, hyperthermia, acute traumatic injuries, and other end-organ damage, should be pursued. Activated charcoal could benefit patients early after ingestion. In the case of PCP, activated charcoal may also decrease gastroenteric recirculation, shortening the effective half-life.[142]

Domoic Acid

Domoic acid is a neurotoxin, structurally similar to glutamic acid, responsible for amnestic shellfish poisoning (ASP). Domoic acid is produced naturally by various strains of phytoplankton, and is subsequently bioconcentrated by shellfish and finfish (cockles, crabs, furrow shell, mussels, razor clams, scallops) before being inadvertently ingested by humans.[143,144] Domoic acid appears to act as a glutamic acid agonist at all 3 ionotropic glutamate receptors (NMDA, 2-amino-3-(5-methyl-3-oxo-1, 2-oxazol-4-yl)propanoic acid [AMPA], kainate).[144] Ingestion produces gastrointestinal symptoms (nausea, vomiting, abdominal cramps, diarrhea) and neurologic complaints (headache, short-term memory loss). Severe poisoning leads to profound neurologic disturbances including hemiparesis, seizures, coma, and autonomic instability.[143] Treatment is supportive.

PERIPHERAL NEUROTOXIC AGENTS

Although both acetylcholine and glycine are well represented in the CNS, many of their xenobiotic interactions produce effects predominantly expressed in the PNS. In this section, the authors discuss xenobiotics producing PNS effects, many of which are naturally occurring toxins and venoms. Sodium channels are critical to the conduction and propagation of action potentials along peripheral nerves. A select group of xenobiotics targeting the sodium channel are addressed in the final section of the article.

Acetylcholine

Similar to the neurotransmitters discussed earlier, acetylcholine is distributed throughout the brain and spinal cord. Unlike many other neurotransmitters, acetylcholine plays a major role in both the CNS and PNS. It is found in both sympathetic and parasympathetic presynaptic ganglia, parasympathetic postganglionic nerves, somatic motor neurons, and at most postganglionic sympathetically innervated sweat glands. Acetylcholine is synthesized by the enzyme choline acetyltransferase and is degraded within the synapse by acetylcholinesterase. A similar enzyme, pseudocholinesterase, is made in the liver and circulates in the plasma. It metabolizes some xenobiotics, like succinylcholine and cocaine, but does not play a large role in the metabolism of acetylcholine.

There are two major types of cholinergic receptors: nicotinic and muscarinic. Nicotinic receptors are ligand-gated ion channels. The receptors at the neuromuscular junction (NMJ nAchR) mediate sodium influx, stimulating depolarization of the endplate and propagation of an action potential down the muscle. Nicotinic receptors at other neuronal sites, both centrally and peripherally, mediate both sodium and calcium influx.[71] Although there are 5 different subtypes of muscarinic acetylcholine receptor, all are G-protein mediated.[73]

The central effects of acetylcholine are primarily mediated by muscarinic receptors because the majority of CNS nicotinic receptors reside in the spinal cord.[71] The central effects are usually accompanied by their corresponding peripheral effects.

Acetylcholine agonism can be produced by direct stimulation of acetylcholine receptors, or by inhibition of acetylcholinesterase (thereby increasing the amounts of acetylcholine within the nerve terminal). Excessive acetylcholine stimulation produces the classic cholinergic syndrome.[145] Central muscarinic effects include sedation, coma, extrapyramidal movement disorders, and seizures. Central nicotinic effects also include seizures. Peripheral muscarinic effects include excessive secretion at salivary, sweat, lacrimal, and bronchial glands, bronchoconstriction, nausea, vomiting, diarrhea, gastrointestinal cramping, urinary incontinence, and fecal incontinence, commonly coined the "SLUDGE" syndrome. Peripheral nicotinic effects include fasciculations, weakness, and flaccid paralysis. Weaponized nerve agents (eg, sarin and VX), organophosphate insecticides, and carbamate insecticides are the prototypical cholinergic agents.

Acetylcholine antagonism produces the collection of symptoms commonly referred to as the anticholinergic syndrome: hyperthermia, tachycardia, flushed skin, anhydrosis, mydriasis, hypoactive bowel sounds, urinary retention, delirium, agitation, picking movements, hallucinations, and coma. The mnemonic "hot as a hare, red as a beet, dry as a bone, blind as a bat, and mad as a hatter" summarizes the progression.[100] These symptoms are mediated predominately through inhibition at muscarinic sites, thus this syndrome is more precisely described as an antimuscarinic syndrome.[71] Hundreds of medications possess antimuscarinic properties, including atropine and other belladonna alkaloids, tricyclic antidepressants, phenothiazine antipsychotics, antiparkinsonian medications, and antihistamines. Natural causes of antimuscarinic poisoning include jimson weed (*Datura stramonium*), Deadly nightshade (*Atropa belladonna*), Angel's trumpet (*Cestrum nocturnum*), Henbane (*Hyoscyamus niger*), and Mandrake (*Mandragora officinarum*).[100]

The NMJ nAchR are a frequent target of xenobiotics that cause peripheral neurotoxic emergencies. The neurotoxic effects are produced in 1 of 3 ways: direct neuromuscular blockade, inhibition of acetylcholine release, or alteration of sodium channel function.

Snake Venom Neurotoxins

Neurotoxins comprise a small proportion of the complex mixture of enzymes, proteins, polypeptides, metals, and various other components in snake venom. The majority of snake neurotoxins cause a progressive generalized flaccid paralysis, initially affecting cranial nerves, with ptosis, ophthalmoplegia, dysarthria, dysphagia, and drooling, then progressing to generalized weakness and finally paralysis of the respiratory muscles.[146] The resultant respiratory paralysis is partially responsible for the estimated 125,000 deaths from snakebite each year.[146] Neuromuscular blockade at the NMJ nAchR is the mechanism by which these neurotoxic venoms exert their effects. Some venom neurotoxins, like those of coral snakes, cobras, and sea snakes, competitively block the NMJ nAchR.[147–150] These effects can be reversed by antivenom or with the administration of an anticholinesterase, such as neostigmine.[147,150] Venom from the Mojave rattlesnake (*Crotalus scutulatus*), and a few other *Crotalus* species, contains a different neurotoxin that inhibits the presynaptic release of acetylcholine from the neuromuscular junction.[148–150] Unless administered early, before the neurotoxin reaches the NMJ, antivenom is unlikely to be beneficial.[146,148] Acetylcholinesterase therapy is unhelpful in these instances.[150]

Tick Paralysis

Once attached a host, the mature female tick secretes a potent neurotoxin causing a slow, ascending, flaccid paralysis. More than 60 different species of tick are associated with tick paralysis. In the United States the most commonly associated species are the wood tick (*Dermacentor andersoni*) and the dog tick (*Dermacentor variabilis*).[151] Similar to the presynaptic snake toxins, the neurotoxin of tick paralysis inhibits the presynaptic release of acetylcholine at the NMJ, causing a symmetric ascending paralysis, and ultimately respiratory muscle failure.[151–153] Removal of the tick leads to gradual recovery, although in some Australian tick species (*Ixodes holocyclus*) recovery may be delayed.[151]

Botulism

Botulism poisoning (*botulus* is latin for sausage) has been well documented since the eighteenth century as a cause of descending flaccid paralysis.[154] Botulinum toxins (BOTOX) are exotoxins of the anaerobic spore-forming bacterium *Clostridium botulinum*. There are 8 different serotypes of *C botulinum*, which make 7 serologically distinct exotoxins (A-G).[155] Similar to tic paralysis and presynaptic snake neurotoxins, BOTOX blocks the release of acetylcholine presynaptically at the NMJ, initially leading to cranial nerve and bulbar symptoms (blurred vision, diplopia, dysarthria, dysphagia, or dysphonia), then progressing to an acute, symmetric, descending motor paralysis with little sensory or autonomic involvement.[154,156,157] BOTOX does not cross the blood-brain barrier, thus there are no central effects.[158]

Humans are exposed to BOTOX in a variety of ways. The most well known, food-borne botulism, occurs after ingestion of food contaminated with the preformed BOTOX. Wound botulism occurs when the spores of *C botulinum* in contaminated wounds germinate and produce BOTOX. The incidence of wound botulism is increasing in heroin addicts who subcutaneously inject black tar heroin ("skin popping").[157] Infant botulism occurs when spores are ingested and subsequently germinate in the infant's immature intestinal tract. Adult intestinal botulism occurs in adults with intestinal flora altered by antibiotic use and other gastrointestinal disorders. Weaponized, aerosolized BOTOX would cause inhalational botulism after release in a bioterrorism attack.[157,159]

Treatment includes vigilant supportive care with close observation for signs of respiratory weakness that might indicate the need for elective intubation and mechanical ventilation. Early antibiotics and surgical debridement are warranted in cases of wound botulism. Definitive treatment with botulinum antitoxin should be given to any patient with a clinical suspicion for botulism. Antitoxin neutralizes free BOTOX in the serum, thus it arrests the progression of symptoms but will not reverse those already present.[158] The standard botulinum antitoxin is horse-derived with antibodies against subtypes A, B, and E. It is obtained by contacting the local or state health department or the Centers for Disease Control and Prevention. BabyBIG is a human-derived immune globulin effective against subtypes A and B, used in the treatment of infant botulism.[157,158] The US Army possesses an antitoxin against all seven serotypes for use in the event of a bioterrorism event.[157,159]

Latrodectism

Widow spiders of the Genus *Latrodectus* are endemic worldwide. The black widow spider, *Latrodectus mactans*, is the most commonly recognized, due to the red hourglass-shaped markings on its ventral abdomen, but other *Latrodectus* species are also endemic in North America. Only the female spider is considered venomous because the smaller male's fangs are not large enough to penetrate human skin. The neurotoxin responsible for latrodectism, α-latrotoxin, facilitates calcium influx into the presynaptic neuron, stimulating massive release of acetylcholine at the neuromuscular junction.[160–162] α-Latrotoxin has similar effects at other peripheral and central acetylcholine and NE neurons as well.[161,163]

Predominant symptoms include muscle pain, spasms, and abdominal rigidity that on occasion has been mistaken for an acute surgical abdomen.[160,162,164] Accompanying symptoms include perspiration, restlessness, anxiety, nausea, vomiting, diarrhea, tachycardia, and hypertension.[162,163] Priapism, facies latrodectismica (facial grimacing), pavor mortis (fear of death), conjunctivitis, and compartment syndrome are less common.[163]

Treatment is supportive with local wound care, tetanus prophylaxis, and the liberal use of opioids and benzodiazepines for relief of pain, anxiety, and muscle spasms. Latrodectus antivenom is rapidly effective but its use is somewhat controversial, due to the very low risk of anaphylaxis and serum sickness. Development of a Fab fragment antivenom is currently under way. Alternative treatments, including calcium gluconate, methocarbamol, and dantrolene, have not proved to be effective.[165,166]

Glycine

Glycine is an inhibitory neurotransmitter found primarily in the spinal cord and lower brainstem, where it plays a large role in mediating motor and sensory reflex circuits.

The glycine receptor is a ligand-gated chloride ion channel receptor similar in structure to the GABA$_A$ receptor.[167]

Strychnine

Strychnine is the natural alkaloid found in the dried seeds of the Southeast Asian tree, *Strychnos nux-vomica*.[168] Strychnine is used as a rodenticide, as a component of some traditional remedies, and as an occasional adulterant in street drugs such as amphetamines, heroin, and cocaine.[168–170] Strychnine is a competitive inhibitor at the glycine receptor. Glycine antagonism leads to uncontrolled muscular activity, initially causing heightened awareness, muscular spasms, and twitches, then progressing to generalized convulsions. The patient remains conscious, afraid, and in pain throughout the course.[168,170] Death is usually caused by respiratory arrest from respiratory muscle spasm. There is no known antidote; treatment is symptomatic and supportive. Benzodiazepines and barbiturates should be used liberally to control muscular spasms. If unsuccessful, nondepolarizing neuromuscular blockade with mechanical ventilation is required. Complications including hypoxia, aspiration, hyperthermia, rhabdomyolysis, and metabolic acidosis should be anticipated.

Tetanus

Tetanus (from the Greek word *tetanos*, to contract) has been known as a disease entity for over 20 centuries.[154] Under favorable anaerobic conditions, the bacillus *Clostridium tetani* produces tetanus toxin. The spores of *C tetani* are ubiquitous in the soil, but more prevalent in soil contaminated by the feces of animals.[171] These spores germinate in dirty wounds, leading to the production of tetanus toxin. Tetanus toxin inhibits the presynaptic release of GABA and glycine in a manner that closely parallels botulism.[154,156,157] There are 4 clinical types of tetanus.[157,171] Generalized tetanus is the most common, causing symptoms strikingly similar to those caused by strychnine. Opisthotonus and risus sardonicus are classically described in patients suffering from tetanus but can be seen in strychnine poisoning as well. With localized tetanus, rigidity and pain remain localized to the site of injury. Cephalic tetanus occurs with injuries to the head or neck and involves the lower cranial nerve musculature. Neonatal tetanus usually follows an umbilical stump infection and may initially present with failure to feed, inability to suck, and weakness. Treatment includes supportive care, wound management, antibiotics, active immunization with a tetanus toxoid–containing vaccine, and passive immunization with tetanus-specific immune globulin.[157,171] Similarly to strychnine, benzodiazepines are first-line agents for control of spasms. Nondepolarizing neuromuscular blockade and mechanical ventilation may be required in severe cases. A high suspicion for complications similar to those of strychnine should be maintained.

Sodium Channels

Just as nicotinic acetylcholine receptors mediate sodium influx through an ion channel, voltage-sensitive sodium ion channels mediate action potential propagation in skeletal muscle, nerve, and cardiac cells.[172] Slight alterations of sodium influx through these channels can easily produce detrimental consequences in membrane excitability. Several xenobiotics induce neurotoxic emergencies in this fashion, by altering sodium entry through these various voltage-sensitive sodium ion channels.

Ciguatera

Ciguatera poisoning is the most commonly reported marine food poisoning. The causative agent, ciguatoxin, is produced by the marine dinoflagellate, *Gambierdiscus toxicus*, and concentrates in the food chain as carnivorous fish eat the smaller herbivorous fish that ingest these dinoflagellates.[173] Humans ingest ciguatoxin when dining on large predatory reef fish including grouper, snapper, barracuda, amberjack, and sea bass.[158] Ciguatoxin binds to voltage-sensitive sodium channels, causing prolonged opening and excitation of skeletal, cardiac, and neuronal tissues.[158,174,175] Ciguatera poisoning leads to 4 categories of symptoms: gastrointestinal (nausea, vomiting, diarrhea), neuropathic (paresthesias, dysthesias, pruritus, diaphoresis, myalgias, arthralgias, weakness), cardiovascular (symptomatic bradycardia), and diffuse pain syndrome. Temperature allodynia (cold reversal, wherein cold items feel hot and possibly vice versa) and the sensation that the teeth are falling out are almost pathognomonic for ciguatera poisoning.[176] Treatment is largely supportive. Although mannitol has been recommended by some investigators, randomized controlled trials have failed to show benefit.[158,174,176]

Neurotoxic Shellfish Poisoning

Neurotoxic shellfish poisoning (NSP) is caused by brevetoxins, a family of toxins that, like ciguatera, open voltage-sensitive sodium channels.[173] The toxin is produced by the dinoflagellate *Kerenia brevis* (formerly *Gymnodinium breve*).[173,175] Brevetoxins are concentrated in filter-feeding shellfish (oysters, clams, coquinas, and other bivalve mollusks).[177] Symptoms are similar to the gastrointestinal and neuropathic symptoms of ciguatera poisoning, but typically resolve within 48 hours.[175] Treatment is supportive.

Poison Dart Frogs

Batrachotoxin is a potent sodium channel opener excreted from the skin of brightly colored *Phyllobates* frogs.[178] These frogs are commonly referred to as "poison dart frogs," presumably referring to the South American Indians' use of their secretions to poison the tips of blowdarts.

Paralytic Shellfish Poisoning

Paralytic shellfish poisoning (PSP) is the most common form of toxin-related disease associated with shellfish ingestion.[177] PSP toxins, saxitoxins, are produced by dinoflagellates of the genera *Alexandrium*. These toxins accumulate in filter-feeding shellfish (mussels, scallops, and clams) similar to NSP, but also have been found in the predators of shellfish, including crustaceans, gastropods, and fish.[175,177,179] Unlike the sodium channel openers discussed above, saxitoxins block voltage-gated sodium channels, preventing the generation of a proper action potential in nerves and muscles.[179] Symptoms include paresthesias, headache, nausea, vomiting, and diarrhea, followed by weakness, dysarthria, and dysphagia. In severe cases weakness progresses to neuromuscular paralysis and respiratory arrest.[175,177,179] Treatment is supportive.

Pufferfish Poisoning

Tetrodotoxin (TTX) is found in a variety of bony fish from the family *Tetraodontidae* including the pufferfish, toad fish, blowfish, balloon fish, and porcupine fish.[177] TTX is also found in a variety of other animals including certain mollusks, the horseshoe crab, the Californian newt, Costa Rican *Atelopus* frogs, and the blue-ringed octopus.[158,180] TTX poisoning is the most common cause of lethal food poisoning, especially in Japan, where pufferfish is consumed as a delicacy.[177] Similar to saxitoxins, TTX blocks voltage-gated sodium channels, preventing nerve conduction.[158,175,177,180] The high fatality rate associated with TTX poisoning led to the development of a clinical grading system.[158,177] Grade 1 includes perioral numbness and paresthesias, with or without gastrointestinal symptoms. Grade 2 involves numbness of the tongue, face, and distal areas, early motor paralysis, uncoordination, and slurred speech. Grade 3 includes generalized flaccid paralysis, respiratory failure, aphonia, and fixed dilated pupils. In grade 4 patients suffer severe respiratory failure with hypoxia, hypotension, bradycardia, and cardiac arrhythmias.[158,177]

Treatment is supportive and focuses on ventilatory support. Lavage and activated charcoal should be considered in those presenting quickly after ingestion. Vasoactive pressor agents and mechanical ventilation may be necessary in moderate to severe cases.

SUMMARY

Acute neurotoxic emergencies manifest with a diverse array of clinical presentations that include drug-induced or toxin-induced seizures, acute excited mental status, acute depressed mental status, and a variety of PNS effects. Understanding the neurotransmitter interactions and pathophysiology of causative xenobiotics helps the provider anticipate the clinical effects of a particular exposure and directs focused therapeutic interventions.

REFERENCES

1. Stedman's medical dictionary. 25th edition. Baltimore(MD): Williams & Wilkins; 1990.
2. Thundiyil JG, Rowley F, Papa L, et al. Risk factors for complications of drug-induced seizures. J Med Toxicol 2011;7:16–23.
3. Thundiyil JG, Kearney TE, Olson KR. Evolving epidemiology of drug-induced seizures reported to a poison control center system. J Toxicol Clin Toxicol 2004;42(5):730.
4. Olson KR, Kearney TE, Dyer JE, et al. Seizures associated with poisoning and drug overdose. Am J Emerg Med 1994;12(3):392–5.
5. Sharma AN, Hoffman RJ. Toxin-related seizures. Emerg Med Clin North Am 2011;29(1):125–39.
6. Woolf AD, Erdman AR, Nelson LS, et al. Tricyclic antidepressant poisoning: an evidence-based consensus guideline for out-of-hospital management. Clin Toxicol (Phila) 2007;45(3):203–33.
7. Bebarta VS, Maddry J, Borys DJ, et al. Incidence of tricyclic antidepressant-like complications after cyclobenzaprine overdose. Am J Emerg Med 2010. [Epub ahead of print].
8. Bradberry SM, Thanacoody HK, Watt BE, et al. Management of the cardiovascular complications of tricyclic antidepressant poisoning: role of sodium bicarbonate. Toxicol Rev 2005;24(3):195–204.
9. Dhillon S, Yang LP, Curran MP. Spotlight on bupropion in major depressive disorder. CNS Drugs 2008;22(7):613–7.
10. Starr P, Klein-Schwartz W, Spiller H, et al. Incidence and onset of delayed seizures after overdoses of extended-release bupropion. Am J Emerg Med 2009; 27(8):911–5.
11. Nelson LS, Erdman AR, Booze LL, et al. Selective serotonin reuptake inhibitor poisoning: an evidence-based consensus guideline for out-of-hospital management. Clin Toxicol (Phila) 2007;45(4):315–32.
12. Waring WS, Gray JA, Graham A. Predictive factors for generalized seizures after deliberate citalopram overdose. Br J Clin Pharmacol 2008;66(6):861–5.

13. Hayes BD, Klein-Schwartz W, Clark RF, et al. Comparison of toxicity of acute overdoses with citalopram and escitalopram. J Emerg Med 2010;39(1):44–8.
14. Yilmaz Z, Ceschi A, Rauber-Luthy C, et al. Escitalopram causes fewer seizures in human overdose than citalopram. Clin Toxicol (Phila) 2010;48(3):207–12.
15. Perucca E, Gram L, Avanzini G, et al. Antiepileptic drugs as a cause of worsening seizures. Epilepsia 1998;39(1):5–17.
16. Spiller HA, Carlisle RD. Status epilepticus after massive carbamazepine overdose. J Toxicol Clin Toxicol 2002;40(1):81–90.
17. Sullivan JB Jr, Rumack BH, Peterson RG. Acute carbamazepine toxicity resulting from overdose. Neurology 1981;31(5):621–4.
18. Guerrini R, Belmonte A, Parmeggiani L, et al. Myoclonic status epilepticus following high-dosage lamotrigine therapy. Brain Dev 1999;21(6):420–4.
19. Hasan M, Lerman-Sagie T, Lev D, et al. Recurrent absence status epilepticus (spike-and-wave stupor) associated with lamotrigine therapy. J Child Neurol 2006;21(9):807–9.
20. Trinka E, Dilitz E, Unterberger I, et al. Non convulsive status epilepticus after replacement of valproate with lamotrigine. J Neurol 2002;249(10):1417–22.
21. Dinnerstein E, Jobst BC, Williamson PD. Lamotrigine intoxication provoking status epilepticus in an adult with localization-related epilepsy. Arch Neurol 2007; 64(9):1344–6.
22. Thundiyil JG, Anderson IB, Stewart PJ, et al. Lamotrigine-induced seizures in a child: case report and literature review. Clin Toxicol (Phila) 2007;45(2): 169–72.
23. Anand JS, Chodorowski Z, Wisniewski M. Seizures induced by topiramate overdose. Clin Toxicol (Phila) 2007;45(2):197.
24. Wisniewski M, Lukasik-Glebocka M, Anand JS. Acute topiramate overdose—clinical manifestations. Clin Toxicol (Phila) 2009;47(4):317–20.
25. Jette N, Cappell J, VanPassel L, et al. Tiagabine-induced nonconvulsive status epilepticus in an adolescent without epilepsy. Neurology 2006;67(8):1514–5.
26. Kazzi ZN, Jones CC, Morgan BW. Seizures in a pediatric patient with a tiagabine overdose. J Med Toxicol 2006;2(4):160–2.
27. Ostrovskiy D, Spanaki MV, Morris GL 3rd. Tiagabine overdose can induce convulsive status epilepticus. Epilepsia 2002;43(7):773–4.
28. Devlin RJ, Henry JA. Clinical review: major consequences of illicit drug consumption. Crit Care 2008;12(1):202.
29. Paloucek FP, Rodvold KA. Evaluation of theophylline overdoses and toxicities. Ann Emerg Med 1988;17(2):135–44.
30. Shanti CM, Lucas CE. Cocaine and the critical care challenge. Crit Care Med 2003;31(6):1851–9.
31. Catravas JD, Waters IW. Acute cocaine intoxication in the conscious dog: studies on the mechanism of lethality. J Pharmacol Exp Ther 1981;217(2):350–6.
32. Gill JR, Hayes JA, deSouza IS, et al. Ecstasy (MDMA) deaths in New York City: a case series and review of the literature. J Forensic Sci 2002;47(1):121–6.
33. Kojima T, Une I, Yashiki M, et al. A fatal methamphetamine poisoning associated with hyperpyrexia. Forensic Sci Int 1984;24(1):87–93.
34. Patel MM, Belson MG, Longwater AB, et al. Methylenedioxymethamphetamine (ecstasy)-related hyperthermia. J Emerg Med 2005;29(4):451–4.
35. Young GP, Rores C, Murphy C, et al. Intravenous phenobarbital for alcohol withdrawal and convulsions. Ann Emerg Med 1987;16(8):847–50.
36. Hyser CL, Drake ME Jr. Status epilepticus after baclofen withdrawal. J Natl Med Assoc 1984;76(5). 533, 537–8.

37. Kofler M, Arturo Leis A. Prolonged seizure activity after baclofen withdrawal. Neurology 1992;42(3 Pt 1):697–8.
38. Peng CT, Ger J, Yang CC, et al. Prolonged severe withdrawal symptoms after acute-on-chronic baclofen overdose. J Toxicol Clin Toxicol 1998;36(4): 359–63.
39. Brust JC. Seizures and substance abuse: treatment considerations. Neurology 2006;67(12 Suppl 4):S45–8.
40. Grond S, Sablotzki A. Clinical pharmacology of tramadol. Clin Pharmacokinet 2004;43(13):879–923.
41. Jovanovic-Cupic V, Martinovic Z, Nesic N. Seizures associated with intoxication and abuse of tramadol. Clin Toxicol (Phila) 2006;44(2):143–6.
42. Shadnia S, Soltaninejad K, Heydari K, et al. Tramadol intoxication: a review of 114 cases. Hum Exp Toxicol 2008;27(3):201–5.
43. Spiller HA, Gorman SE, Villalobos D, et al. Prospective multicenter evaluation of tramadol exposure. J Toxicol Clin Toxicol 1997;35(4):361–4.
44. Afshari R, Ghooshkhanehee H. Tramadol overdose induced seizure, dramatic rise of CPK and acute renal failure. J Pak Med Assoc 2009;59(3):178.
45. Sansone RA, Sansone LA. Tramadol: seizures, serotonin syndrome, and coad-ministered antidepressants. Psychiatry (Edgmont) 2009;6(4):17–21.
46. Lawson AA, Northridge DB. Dextropropoxyphene overdose. Epidemiology, clinical presentation and management. Med Toxicol Adverse Drug Exp 1987;2(6): 430–44.
47. Sloth Madsen P, Strom J, Reiz S, et al. Acute propoxyphene self-poisoning in 222 consecutive patients. Acta Anaesthesiol Scand 1984;28(6):661–5.
48. Stork CM, Redd JT, Fine K, et al. Propoxyphene-induced wide QRS complex dysrhythmia responsive to sodium bicarbonate—a case report. J Toxicol Clin Toxicol 1995;33(2):179–83.
49. Ramirez J, Innocenti F, Schuetz EG, et al. CYP2B6, CYP3A4, and CYP2C19 are responsible for the in vitro N-demethylation of meperidine in human liver microsomes. Drug Metab Dispos 2004;32(9):930–6.
50. Seifert CF, Kennedy S. Meperidine is alive and well in the new millennium: evaluation of meperidine usage patterns and frequency of adverse drug reactions. Pharmacotherapy 2004;24(6):776–83.
51. Maw G, Aitken P. Isoniazid overdose: a case series, literature review and survey of antidote availability. Clin Drug Investig 2003;23(7):479–85.
52. Vale JA, Kulig K. Position paper: gastric lavage. J Toxicol Clin Toxicol 2004; 42(7):933–43.
53. Chyka PA, Seger D, Krenzelok EP, et al. Position paper: single-dose activated charcoal. Clin Toxicol (Phila) 2005;43(2):61–87.
54. Position paper: whole bowel irrigation. J Toxicol Clin Toxicol 2004;42(6):843–54.
55. Bryant SM, Weiselberg R, Metz J, et al. Should no bowel irrigation be a higher priority than whole bowel irrigation in the treatment of sustained-release ingestions? [abstract]. Clin Toxicol (Phila) 2008;47(7):638.
56. Position statement and practice guidelines on the use of multi-dose activated charcoal in the treatment of acute poisoning. American Academy of Clinical Toxicology; European Association of Poisons Centres and Clinical Toxicologists. J Toxicol Clin Toxicol 1999;37(6):731–51.
57. Proudfoot AT, Krenzelok EP, Vale JA. Position paper on urine alkalinization. J Toxicol Clin Toxicol 2004;42(1):1–26.
58. Wills B, Erickson T. Chemically induced seizures. Clin Lab Med 2006;26(1): 185–209, ix.

59. Nolop KB, Natow A. Unprecedented sedative requirements during delirium tremens. Crit Care Med 1985;13(4):246–7.

60. Woo E, Greenblatt DJ. Massive benzodiazepine requirements during acute alcohol withdrawal. Am J Psychiatry 1979;136(6):821–3.

61. Coomes TR, Smith SW. Successful use of propofol in refractory delirium tremens. Ann Emerg Med 1997;30(6):825–8.

62. McCowan C, Marik P. Refractory delirium tremens treated with propofol: a case series. Crit Care Med 2000;28(6):1781–4.

63. Claassen J, Hirsch LJ, Emerson RG, et al. Treatment of refractory status epilepticus with pentobarbital, propofol, or midazolam: a systematic review. Epilepsia 2002;43(2):146–53.

64. Rossetti AO, Reichhart MD, Schaller MD, et al. Propofol treatment of refractory status epilepticus: a study of 31 episodes. Epilepsia 2004;45(7):757–63.

65. Shah AS, Eddleston M. Should phenytoin or barbiturates be used as second-line anticonvulsant therapy for toxicological seizures? Clin Toxicol (Phila) 2010;48(8):800–5.

66. Bazil CW, Pedley TA. Clinical pharmacology of antiepileptic drugs. Clin Neuropharmacol 2003;26(1):38–52.

67. Tutka P, Mroz T, Klucha K, et al. Bupropion-induced convulsions: preclinical evaluation of antiepileptic drugs. Epilepsy Res 2005;64(1/2):13–22.

68. Brent J, Vo N, Kulig K, et al. Reversal of prolonged isoniazid-induced coma by pyridoxine. Arch Intern Med 1990;150(8):1751–3.

69. Shannon M, McElroy EA, Liebelt EL. Toxic seizures in children: case scenarios and treatment strategies. Pediatr Emerg Care 2003;19(3):206–10.

70. Uusi-Oukari M, Korpi ER. Regulation of GABA(A) receptor subunit expression by pharmacological agents. Pharmacol Rev 2010;62(1):97–135.

71. Curry SC, Mills KC, Ruha AM, et al. Neurotransmitters and neuromodulators. In: Nelson LS, Lewin NA, Howland MA, et al, editors. Goldfrank's toxicologic emergencies. 9th edition. New York: McGraw-Hill Companies; 2011. p. 189–220.

72. Bormann J. The 'ABC' of GABA receptors. Trends Pharmacol Sci 2000;21(1):16–9.

73. Akhtar J, Rittenberger JC. Clinical neurotoxicology. In: Shannon MW, Borron SW, Burns MJ, editors. Haddad and Winchester's clinical management of poisoning and drug overdose. 4th edition. Philadelphia: Elsevier; 2007. p. 191–207.

74. Korpi ER, Mattila MJ, Wisden W, et al. GABA(A)-receptor subtypes: clinical efficacy and selectivity of benzodiazepine site ligands. Ann Med 1997;29(4):275–82.

75. Luddens H, Korpi ER, Seeburg PH. GABA$_A$/benzodiazepine receptor heterogeneity: neurophysiological implications. Neuropharmacology 1995;34(3):245–54.

76. Olsen RW, Li GD. GABA(A) receptors as molecular targets of general anesthetics: identification of binding sites provides clues to allosteric modulation. Can J Anaesth 2011;58(2):206–15.

77. Halpern JH. Hallucinogens and dissociative agents naturally growing in the United States. Pharmacol Ther 2004;102(2):131–8.

78. Shirley KW, Kothare S, Piatt JH Jr, et al. Intrathecal baclofen overdose and withdrawal. Pediatr Emerg Care 2006;22(4):258–61.

79. Chateauvieux S, Morceau F, Dicato M, et al. Molecular and therapeutic potential and toxicity of valproic acid. J Biomed Biotechnol 2010;2010:479364.

80. Mesdjian E, Ciesielski L, Valli M, et al. Sodium valproate: kinetic profile and effects on GABA levels in various brain areas of the rat. Prog Neuropsychopharmacol Biol Psychiatry 1982;6(3):223–33.

81. Urban MO, Ren K, Park KT, et al. Comparison of the antinociceptive profiles of gabapentin and 3-methylgabapentin in rat models of acute and persistent pain: implications for mechanism of action. J Pharmacol Exp Ther 2005;313(3): 1209–16.

82. Sarup A, Larsson OM, Schousboe A. GABA transporters and GABA-transaminase as drug targets. Curr Drug Targets CNS Neurol Disord 2003;2(4): 269–77.

83. McNamara JO. Pharmacotherapy of the epilepsies. In: Brunton LL, Lazo JS, Parker KL, editors. Goodman & Gillman's the pharmacological basis of therapeutics. 11th edition. New York: Mc-Graw Hill; 2005. p. 501–25.

84. Ngo AS, Anthony CR, Samuel M, et al. Should a benzodiazepine antagonist be used in unconscious patients presenting to the emergency department? Resuscitation 2007;74(1):27–37.

85. Seger DL. Flumazenil—treatment or toxin. J Toxicol Clin Toxicol 2004;42(2): 209–16.

86. Nemeth Z, Kun B, Demetrovics Z. The involvement of gamma-hydroxybutyrate in reported sexual assaults: a systematic review. J Psychopharmacol 2010; 24(9):1281–7.

87. Carter LP, Koek W, France CP. Behavioral analyses of GHB: receptor mechanisms. Pharmacol Ther 2009;121(1):100–14.

88. Maitre M. The gamma-hydroxybutyrate signalling system in brain: organization and functional implications. Prog Neurobiol 1997;51(3):337–61.

89. Wong CG, Gibson KM, Snead OC 3rd. From the street to the brain: neurobiology of the recreational drug gamma-hydroxybutyric acid. Trends Pharmacol Sci 2004;25(1):29–34.

90. Li J, Stokes SA, Woeckener A. A tale of novel intoxication: a review of the effects of gamma-hydroxybutyric acid with recommendations for management. Ann Emerg Med 1998;31(6):729–36.

91. Liechti ME, Kunz I, Greminger P, et al. Clinical features of gamma-hydroxybutyrate and gamma-butyrolactone toxicity and concomitant drug and alcohol use. Drug Alcohol Depend 2006;81(3):323–6.

92. Zvosec DL, Smith SW, McCutcheon JR, et al. Adverse events, including death, associated with the use of 1,4-butanediol. N Engl J Med 2001;344(2): 87–94.

93. Shannon M, Quang LS. Gamma-hydroxybutyrate, gamma-butyrolactone, and 1,4-butanediol: a case report and review of the literature. Pediatr Emerg Care 2000;16(6):435–40.

94. Van Sassenbroeck DK, De Neve N, De Paepe P, et al. Abrupt awakening phenomenon associated with gamma-hydroxybutyrate use: a case series. Clin Toxicol (Phila) 2007;45(5):533–8.

95. Farmer BM. Gamma-hydroxybutyric acid. In: Nelson LS, Lewin NA, Howland MA, et al, editors. Goldfrank's toxicologic emergencies. 9th edition. New York: McGraw Hill; 2011. p. 1151–6.

96. Quang LS. GHB and related compounds. In: Shannon MW, Borron SW, Burns MJ, editors. Haddad and Winchester's clinical management of poisoning and drug overdose. 4th edition. Philadelphia: Elsevier; 2007. p. 803–23.

97. LeTourneau JL, Hagg DS, Smith SM. Baclofen and gamma-hydroxybutyrate withdrawal. Neurocrit Care 2008;8(3):430–3.

98. Trescot AM, Datta S, Lee M, et al. Opioid pharmacology. Pain Physician 2008; 11(Suppl 2):S133–53.

99. Dietis N, Guerrini R, Calo G, et al. Simultaneous targeting of multiple opioid receptors: a strategy to improve side-effect profile. Br J Anaesth 2009;103(1): 38–49.
100. Meehan TJ, Bryant SM, Aks SE. Drugs of abuse: the highs and lows of altered mental states in the emergency department. Emerg Med Clin North Am 2010; 28(3):663–82.
101. Dahan A, Aarts L, Smith TW. Incidence, reversal, and prevention of opioid-induced respiratory depression. Anesthesiology 2010;112(1):226–38.
102. Vardakou I, Pistos C, Spiliopoulou C. Spice drugs as a new trend: mode of action, identification and legislation. Toxicol Lett 2010;197(3):157–62.
103. Schneir AB, Cullen J, Ly BT. "Spice" girls: synthetic cannabinoid intoxication. J Emerg Med 2011;40(3):296–9.
104. Elkashef A, Vocci F, Huestis M, et al. Marijuana neurobiology and treatment. Subst Abus 2008;29(3):17–29.
105. Felder CC, Glass M. Cannabinoid receptors and their endogenous agonists. Annu Rev Pharmacol Toxicol 1998;38:179–200.
106. McPartland JM. The endocannabinoid system: an osteopathic perspective. J Am Osteopath Assoc 2008;108(10):586–600.
107. Ashton CH. Pharmacology and effects of cannabis: a brief review. Br J Psychiatry 2001;178:101–6.
108. Iversen L. Cannabis and the brain. Brain 2003;126(Pt 6):1252–70.
109. Campbell FA, Tramer MR, Carroll D, et al. Are cannabinoids an effective and safe treatment option in the management of pain? A qualitative systematic review. BMJ 2001;323(7303):13–6.
110. Johns A. Psychiatric effects of cannabis. Br J Psychiatry 2001;178:116–22.
111. Every-Palmer S. Synthetic cannabinoid JWH-018 and psychosis: an explorative study. Drug Alcohol Depend 2011. [Epub ahead of print].
112. Zimmermann US, Winkelmann PR, Pilhatsch M, et al. Withdrawal phenomena and dependence syndrome after the consumption of "spice gold". Dtsch Arztebl Int 2009;106(27):464–7.
113. Insel PA. Seminars in medicine of the Beth Israel Hospital, Boston. Adrenergic receptors—evolving concepts and clinical implications. N Engl J Med 1996; 334(9):580–5.
114. Beaulieu JM, Gainetdinov RR. The physiology, signaling, and pharmacology of dopamine receptors. Pharmacol Rev 2011;63(1):182–217.
115. Millan MJ, Marin P, Bockaert J, et al. Signaling at G-protein-coupled serotonin receptors: recent advances and future research directions. Trends Pharmacol Sci 2008;29(9):454–64.
116. Green AR, Mechan AO, Elliott JM, et al. The pharmacology and clinical pharmacology of 3,4-methylenedioxymethamphetamine (MDMA, "ecstasy"). Pharmacol Rev 2003;55(3):463–508.
117. Sulzer D, Sonders MS, Poulsen NW, et al. Mechanisms of neurotransmitter release by amphetamines: a review. Prog Neurobiol 2005;75(6):406–33.
118. Aghajanian GK, Marek GJ. Serotonin and hallucinogens. Neuropsychopharmacology 1999;21(Suppl 2):16S–23S.
119. DEA. Methylenedioxypyrovalerone (MDPV). Drugs and chemicals of concern. 2011. Available at: http://www.deadiversion.usdoj.gov/drugs_concern/mdpv.pdf. Accessed March 26, 2011.
120. ACMD. Consideration of the cathinones. Advisory council on the misuse of drugs. 2010. Available at: http://www.namsdl.org/documents/ACMDCathinonesReport. pdf. Accessed March 26, 2011.

121. Schwartz BG, Rezkalla S, Kloner RA. Cardiovascular effects of cocaine. Circulation 2010;122(24):2558–69.
122. Smith JA, Mo Q, Guo H, et al. Cocaine increases extraneuronal levels of aspartate and glutamate in the nucleus accumbens. Brain Res 1995;683(2): 264–9.
123. Guidelines 2000 for cardiopulmonary resuscitation and emergency cardiovascular care. Part 8: advanced challenges in resuscitation: section 2: toxicology in ECC. The American Heart Association in collaboration with the International Liaison Committee on Resuscitation. Circulation 2000;102(Suppl 8): I223–8.
124. Albertson TE, Dawson A, de Latorre F, et al. TOX-ACLS: toxicologic-oriented advanced cardiac life support. Ann Emerg Med 2001;37(Suppl 4):S78–90.
125. Lange RA, Cigarroa RG, Flores ED, et al. Potentiation of cocaine-induced coronary vasoconstriction by beta-adrenergic blockade. Ann Intern Med 1990; 112(12):897–903.
126. Boyer EW, Shannon M. The serotonin syndrome. N Engl J Med 2005;352(11): 1112–20.
127. Juurlink DN. Antipsychotics. In: Nelson LS, Lewin NA, Howland MA, et al, editors. Goldfrank's toxicologic emergencies. 9th edition. New York: McGraw Hill; 2011. p. 1103–15.
128. Levine M, Burns MJ. Antipsychotic agents. In: Shannon MW, Borron SW, Burns MJ, editors. Haddad and Winchester's clinical management of poisoning and drug overdose. 4th edition. Philadelphia: Elsevier; 2007. p. 703–20.
129. Adnet P, Lestavel P, Krivosic-Horber R. Neuroleptic malignant syndrome. Br J Anaesth 2000;85(1):129–35.
130. Strawn JR, Keck PE Jr, Caroff SN. Neuroleptic malignant syndrome. Am J Psychiatry 2007;164(6):870–6.
131. Reulbach U, Dutsch C, Biermann T, et al. Managing an effective treatment for neuroleptic malignant syndrome. Crit Care 2007;11(1):R4.
132. Ener RA, Meglathery SB, Van Decker WA, et al. Serotonin syndrome and other serotonergic disorders. Pain Med 2003;4(1):63–74.
133. Birmes P, Coppin D, Schmitt L, et al. Serotonin syndrome: a brief review. CMAJ 2003;168(11):1439–42.
134. Isbister GK, Buckley NA. The pathophysiology of serotonin toxicity in animals and humans: implications for diagnosis and treatment. Clin Neuropharmacol 2005;28(5):205–14.
135. Radomski JW, Dursun SM, Reveley MA, et al. An exploratory approach to the serotonin syndrome: an update of clinical phenomenology and revised diagnostic criteria. Med Hypotheses 2000;55(3):218–24.
136. Javitt DC. Glutamate as a therapeutic target in psychiatric disorders. Mol Psychiatry 2004;9(11):984–97, 979.
137. Kew JN, Kemp JA. Ionotropic and metabotropic glutamate receptor structure and pharmacology. Psychopharmacology (Berl) 2005;179(1):4–29.
138. Mori H, Mishina M. Structure and function of the NMDA receptor channel. Neuropharmacology 1995;34(10):1219–37.
139. Weiner AL, Vieira L, McKay CA, et al. Ketamine abusers presenting to the emergency department: a case series. J Emerg Med 2000;18(4):447–51.
140. Bahn EL, Holt KR. Procedural sedation and analgesia: a review and new concepts. Emerg Med Clin North Am 2005;23(2):503–17.
141. Reich DL, Silvay G. Ketamine: an update on the first twenty-five years of clinical experience. Can J Anaesth 1989;36(2):186–97.

142. Liang IE, Boyer EW. Dissociative agents: phencyclidine, ketamine and dextromethorphan. In: Shannon MW, Borron SW, Burns MJ, editors. Haddad and Winchester's clinical management of poisoning and drug overdose. 4th edition. Philadelphia: Elsevier; 2007. p. 773–9.
143. Jeffery B, Barlow T, Moizer K, et al. Amnesic shellfish poison. Food Chem Toxicol 2004;42(4):545–57.
144. Lefebvre KA, Robertson A. Domoic acid and human exposure risks: a review. Toxicon 2010;56(2):218–30.
145. Sidell FR, Borak J. Chemical warfare agents: II. Nerve agents. Ann Emerg Med 1992;21(7):865–71.
146. White J, Warrell D, Eddleston M, et al. Clinical toxinology—where are we now? J Toxicol Clin Toxicol 2003;41(3):263–76.
147. Khandelwal G, Katz KD, Brooks DE, et al. Naja Kaouthia: two cases of Asiatic cobra envenomations. J Emerg Med 2007;32(2):171–4.
148. Prasarnpun S, Walsh J, Awad SS, et al. Envenoming bites by kraits: the biological basis of treatment-resistant neuromuscular paralysis. Brain 2005;128(Pt 12): 2987–96.
149. Rowan EG. What does beta-bungarotoxin do at the neuromuscular junction? Toxicon 2001;39(1):107–18.
150. Sanmuganathan PS. Myasthenic syndrome of snake envenomation: a clinical and neurophysiological study. Postgrad Med J 1998;74(876):596–9.
151. Edlow JA, McGillicuddy DC. Tick paralysis. Infect Dis Clin North Am 2008;22(3): 397–413, vii.
152. Felz MW, Smith CD, Swift TR. A six-year-old girl with tick paralysis. N Engl J Med 2000;342(2):90–4.
153. Greenstein P. Tick paralysis. Med Clin North Am 2002;86(2):441–6.
154. Humeau Y, Doussau F, Grant NJ, et al. How botulinum and tetanus neurotoxins block neurotransmitter release. Biochimie 2000;82(5):427–46.
155. Klein AW. Complications and adverse reactions with the use of botulinum toxin. Semin Cutan Med Surg 2001;20(2):109–20.
156. Caleo M, Schiavo G. Central effects of tetanus and botulinum neurotoxins. Toxicon 2009;54(5):593–9.
157. Goonetilleke A, Harris JB. Clostridial neurotoxins. J Neurol Neurosurg Psychiatry 2004;75(Suppl 3):iii35–9.
158. Lawrence DT, Dobmeier SG, Bechtel LK, et al. Food poisoning [abstract ix]. Emerg Med Clin North Am 2007;25(2):357–73.
159. Arnon SS, Schechter R, Inglesby TV, et al. Botulinum toxin as a biological weapon: medical and public health management. JAMA 2001;285(8):1059–70.
160. Handel CC, Izquierdo LA, Curet LB. Black widow spider (*Latrodectus mactans*) bite during pregnancy. West J Med 1994;160(3):261–2.
161. Ushkaryov YA, Volynski KE, Ashton AC. The multiple actions of black widow spider toxins and their selective use in neurosecretion studies. Toxicon 2004;43(5): 527–42.
162. Vetter RS, Isbister GK. Medical aspects of spider bites. Annu Rev Entomol 2008; 53:409–29.
163. Graudins A. Spiders. In: Shannon MW, Borron SW, Burns MJ, editors. Haddad and Winchester's clinical management of poisoning and drug overdose. 4th edition. Philadelphia: Elsevier; 2007. p. 433–9.
164. Hahn I. Arthropods. In: Nelson LS, Lewin NA, Howland MA, et al, editors. Goldfrank's toxicologic emergencies. 9th edition. New York: McGraw Hill; 2011. p. 1561–81.

165. Daly FF, Hill RE, Bogdan GM, et al. Neutralization of *Latrodectus mactans* and *L. hesperus* venom by redback spider (*L. hasseltii*) antivenom. J Toxicol Clin Toxicol 2001;39(2):119–23.

166. Isbister GK, Graudins A, White J, et al. Antivenom treatment in arachnidism. J Toxicol Clin Toxicol 2003;41(3):291–300.

167. Webb TI, Lynch JW. Molecular pharmacology of the glycine receptor chloride channel. Curr Pharm Des 2007;13(23):2350–67.

168. Makarovsky I, Markel G, Hoffman A, et al. Strychnine—a killer from the past. Isr Med Assoc J 2008;10(2):142–5.

169. Chan TY. Herbal medicine causing likely strychnine poisoning. Hum Exp Toxicol 2002;21(8):467–8.

170. Wood D, Webster E, Martinez D, et al. Case report: survival after deliberate strychnine self-poisoning, with toxicokinetic data. Crit Care 2002;6(5):456–9.

171. Afshar M, Raju M, Ansell D, et al. Narrative review: tetanus—a health threat after natural disasters in developing countries. Ann Intern Med 2011;154(5):329–35.

172. Wang SY, Wang GK. Voltage-gated sodium channels as primary targets of diverse lipid-soluble neurotoxins. Cell Signal 2003;15(2):151–9.

173. Wang DZ. Neurotoxins from marine dinoflagellates: a brief review. Mar Drugs 2008;6(2):349–71.

174. Purcell CE, Capra MF, Cameron J. Action of mannitol in ciguatoxin-intoxicated rats. Toxicon 1999;37(1):67–76.

175. Sobel J, Painter J. Illnesses caused by marine toxins. Clin Infect Dis 2005;41(9):1290–6.

176. Schnorf H, Taurarii M, Cundy T. Ciguatera fish poisoning: a double-blind randomized trial of mannitol therapy. Neurology 2002;58(6):873–80.

177. Isbister GK. Marine envenomation and poisoning. In: Dart RC, editor. Medical toxicology. 3rd edition. Philadelphia: Lippincott Williams & Wilkins; 2004. p. 1621–44.

178. Bosmans F, Maertens C, Verdonck F, et al. The poison dart frog's batrachotoxin modulates Nav1.8. FEBS Lett 2004;577(1–2):245–8.

179. Araoz R, Molgo J, Tandeau de Marsac N. Neurotoxic cyanobacterial toxins. Toxicon 2010;56(5):813–28.

180. How CK, Chern CH, Huang YC, et al. Tetrodotoxin poisoning. Am J Emerg Med 2003;21(1):51–4.

Antidepressant Overdose–induced Seizures

Bryan S. Judge, MD[a,b,c,*], Landen L. Rentmeester, MD[a,b]

KEYWORDS

- Antidepressants • Overdose • Seizures • Deliberate self-poisoning

COMMENTARY ON ANTIDEPRESSANT OVERDOSE-INDUCED SEIZURES FOR PSYCHIATRIC PRACTICE

Treating patients with psychiatric problems can present numerous challenges for clinicians. The deliberate self-ingestion of antidepressants is one such challenge frequently encountered in hospitals throughout the United States. Since seizures are a serious complication of antidepressant overdose, psychiatrists should be aware of the risk associated with overdose of numerous antidepressants.

This review focuses on (1) the classes of antidepressants, their pharmacologic properties, and some of the proposed mechanism(s) for antidepressant overdose-induced seizures, (2) the evidence for seizures caused by antidepressants in overdose, and (3) management strategies for patients who have intentionally or unintentionally overdosed on an antidepressant, or who have experienced an antidepressant overdose-induced seizure.

This article originally appeared in the *August 2011 issue of Neurologic Clinics (Volume 29, Number 3)*.

The authors have no conflicts, financial or otherwise, to disclose.

[a] Grand Rapids Medical Education Partners/Michigan State University Emergency Medicine Residency, 100 Michigan NE, MC 49, Grand Rapids, MI 49403, USA; [b] Division of Emergency Medicine, Michigan State University College of Human Medicine, 15 Michigan Street NE, Suite 425, Grand Rapids, MI 49503, USA; [c] Spectrum Health-Toxicology Services, 1900 Wealthy Street SE, Suite 255, Grand Rapids, MI 49506, USA

* Corresponding author. Spectrum Health-Toxicology Services, 1900 Wealthy Street SE, Suite 255, Grand Rapids, MI 49506.

E-mail address: bryan.judge@spectrum-health.org

KEY POINTS

Essential points for psychiatric practice in antidepressant overdose-induced seizures include the following:

- Recognizing the seizure risk associated with various antidepressants.
- Understanding the mechanism(s) underlying antidepressant overdose-induced seizures.
- Knowing approaches to treatment for patients who have experienced an antidepressant overdose-induced seizure.

Awareness of the seizure potential of antidepressants in overdose can help determine the need for and duration of inpatient monitoring, and assist in the clinical decision making of physicians caring for these patients.

Human exposure to antidepressants in the United States has rapidly escalated in recent years. Although millions of Americans therapeutically take this class of neuroactive drugs on a daily basis,[1] exposures can also occur after an accidental ingestion or from an intentional overdose. In 2009, antidepressants as a class ranked seventh (n = 102,792) among substance categories most frequently involved in human exposures reported to the National Poison Data System (NPDS).[2] Regardless of the intent of the exposure, antidepressants can result in seizures.[3] Although seizures associated with the therapeutic use of antidepressants are infrequent, their risk after overdose is much greater.[4] Furthermore, antidepressant overdose–induced seizures can generate dilemmas for the clinician such as treating status epilepticus,[5] or determining the need for, and duration of, inpatient monitoring.

Because antidepressant use among patients is common, and because they are frequently involved in intentional and unintentional overdoses, it would benefit practitioners to (1) recognize the seizure propensity associated with various antidepressants, (2) understand the mechanism(s) underlying antidepressant overdose–induced seizures, and (3) be familiar with treatment strategies for patients who have experienced an antidepressant overdose–induced seizure. Therefore, the focus of this review is threefold. First, the classes of antidepressants, their pharmacologic properties, along with some of the proposed mechanism(s) for seizures triggered by antidepressants in overdose, are discussed briefly. Second, pertinent evidence for antidepressant overdose–induced seizures is examined and, after careful scrutiny of this evidence, antidepressants are ranked as high risk (seizure incidence >10% after overdose), intermediate risk (seizure incidence 5%–10% after overdose), or low risk (seizure incidence <5% after overdose) for seizure potential. In addition, management strategies are provided for patients who have intentionally or unintentionally overdosed on an antidepressant, or who have experienced an antidepressant overdose–induced seizure.

PATHOPHYSIOLOGY OF SEIZURE ACTIVITY

Before discussing the various antidepressant classes and the mechanism(s) that may be responsible for antidepressant overdose–induced seizures, it is paramount to briefly review the pathways by which seizures can be triggered. In general, neuronal excitation results from an influx of sodium or diminishment of either chloride conduction or potassium efflux through ion channels. Conversely, neuronal inhibition occurs after a decrease in sodium influx or augmentation of either chloride conduction or potassium efflux through ion channels. When there is gross imbalance between neuronal excitation and inhibition, electrical activity within the central nervous system (CNS) becomes frenzied, and seizures ensue.[6]

There are numerous neurochemical pathways recognized for triggering seizures. Drugs that antagonize adenosine (A_1), histamine (H_1), and γ-aminobutyric acid (GABA) receptors can result in seizures,[7–9] and substances that stimulate cholinergic and glutamatergic receptors can trigger seizures.[10,11] The role of sodium channels in the development and treatment of seizures is complex; although drugs that block sodium channels are often used to prevent seizures (eg, phenytoin), this same mechanism can cause seizures such as those seen with excessive doses of lidocaine.[12] This exemplifies the complex nature underlying the cause and treatment of seizures. Numerous metabolic disturbances can produce seizures: hypocalcemia, hypoglycemia, hyperglycemia, hypomagnesemia, and hyponatremia.[6] Contrary to prior dogma, a solid body of evidence now supports the concept that the noradrenergic and serotonergic effects of antidepressants are anticonvulsant with therapeutic doses, whereas larger doses, such as those that occur with supratherapeutic exposure or an intentional overdose, activate other neurochemical pathways that can culminate in seizures.[13,14]

CLASSIFICATION OF ANTIDEPRESSANTS
Monoamine Oxidase Inhibitors (Isocarboxazid, Moclobemide, Phenelzine, Selegiline, Tranylcypromine)

Monoamine oxidase inhibitors (MAOI) were the first drugs used to treat depression, and were once considered first-line pharmacologic therapy. There are several drugs in this class; however, only a few are used today in the United States for the treatment of refractory depression; these include isocarboxazid, phenelzine, selegiline (transdermal system), and tranylcypromine.[15] Currently, moclobemide is approved as an antidepressant in several countries worldwide but has not been approved for use in the United States.[16]

The primary pharmacologic mechanism by which MAOIs work is the inhibition of the enzyme monoamine oxidase located on the outer mitochondrial membrane of neurons.[17] Consequently, the breakdown of the biogenic amines dopamine, norepinephrine, and serotonin is prevented, thereby increasing the concentration of these neurotransmitters available for reuptake, storage, and subsequent release by neurons.[18] Isocarboxazid, phenelzine, and tranylcypromine are irreversible and nonselective MAOIs; selegiline irreversibly and selectively inhibits monoamine oxidase B; and moclobemide reversibly and selectively inhibits monoamine oxidase A.[16]

Although moclobemide may possess anticonvulsant properties,[19] there is potential for CNS excitation with overdose of the hydrazine derivatives isocarboxazid and phenelzine, and the amphetamine derivative tranylcypromine. Hydrazine derivatives including the antitubercular agent isoniazid diminish the synthesis of GABA in the CNS by antagonizing pyridoxine.[20] The net effect is loss of the normal neural inhibition mediated by GABA, resulting in seizures that are refractory unless treated with pyridoxine. In addition, isocarboxazid and tranylcypromine have been shown to block $GABA_A$ receptors in an animal model[21] and MAOIs may augment CNS excitation by increasing concentrations of neuronal glutamic acid.[22]

Cyclic Antidepressants (Tertiary Amines: Amitriptyline, Clomipramine, Doxepin, Imipramine, Trimipramine. Secondary Amines: Desipramine, Nortriptyline, Protriptyline. Other: Amoxapine, Maprotiline)

Although there has been a substantial decline in the number of people treated with cyclic antidepressants (CAs) in the United States,[1] poisoning and death from the intentional ingestions of this class of antidepressants remains problematic. In 2009, CAs comprised 11.6% (n = 11,873) of human exposures to antidepressants registered with the NPDS, and this substance category tied for 10th place among other substance categories associated with the largest number of fatalities.[2] Cyclic antidepressants can be classified into tertiary amines, which include amitriptyline, clomipramine, doxepin, imipramine, and trimipramine, and secondary amines, which include desipramine, nortriptyline, and protriptyline. Structurally, secondary amines differ from tertiary amines in that they lack a methyl group on the terminal nitrogen of their side chains. The dibenzoxapine CA amoxapine and the tetracyclic antidepressant maprotiline are discussed separately later.

The CAs have a multitude of pharmacologic actions. Their therapeutic effect is primarily mediated through the inhibition of the reuptake of the biogenic amines norepinephrine and serotonin.[23] Toxicity associated with CAs is caused by antagonism of α_1-adrenergic, H_1 histamine, and muscarinic receptors; blockade of cardiac ion channels (Na^+ and K^+); and interference with chloride conductance through GABA Cl^- ionophores.[6,24] Each drug within this class shows variability in these pharmacologic mechanisms of action and their toxic effects. Seizures after a CA overdose are believed to occur secondary to their interference with the influx of chloride through GABA Cl^- channels; these drugs bind to the picrotoxin site on the GABA-chloride complex,[21] but other potential mechanisms include an inhibitory effect on G-protein-activated inwardly rectifying K^+ (GIRK) channels or antagonism of H_1 receptors.[13]

Amoxapine

Introduced in 1980, amoxapine was initially promoted as having a faster onset of antidepressant effects compared with other available CAs.[25] Amoxapine inhibits the reuptake of norepinephrine, moderately antagonizes α_1-adrenergic and D_2 dopamine receptors, and weakly blocks H_1 receptors.[24] Seizure activity is one of the most common adverse reactions reported with amoxapine. Data from the World Health Organization's adverse drug reaction database from 1968 to 2006 noted 121 cases of convulsions out of 1384 reported adverse reactions.[26] Although these data are limited because the total number of patients taking amoxapine in this time period is not known, the percentage of adverse reactions reported as seizures for amoxapine (8.74%) was second only to maprotiline (14.43%) among the CAs. As with other antidepressants, the precise mechanism behind the proconvulsant effect of amoxapine is not fully understood.

Maprotiline

Similar to amoxapine, maprotiline inhibits the reuptake of norepinephrine, and moderately antagonizes α_1-adrenergic receptors, but differs in that it strongly blocks H_1 receptors and weakly antagonizes D_2 and muscarinic receptors.[24] This CA was initially believed to have a safer side effect profile compared with other CAs. However, even with therapeutic use, seizures have been an issue, and the risk for seizures seems to be dose-dependent.[27] One retrospective study found a seizure rate of 15.6% in patients taking between 75 and 300 mg daily.[28] Although it is uncertain what mechanism(s) are responsible for maprotiline-induced seizures, two possibilities include the inhibitory effect that maprotiline exerts on GIRK channels and antagonism of H_1 receptors.[13]

Selective Serotonin Reuptake Inhibitors (Citalopram, Escitalopram, Fluoxetine, Fluvoxamine, Paroxetine, Sertraline)

Because of their tolerability and relative safety in overdose compared with CAs, selective serotonin reuptake inhibitors (SSRIs) have been the preferred class of antidepressants to treat depression since the 1990s.[29] Several SSRIs are available, including citalopram, escitalopram, fluoxetine, fluvoxamine, paroxetine, and sertraline. The pharmacologic mechanism of action for this class of antidepressants is the selective inhibition of serotonin reuptake at the neuronal synapse. In addition, drugs in this class have many other pharmacologic properties: citalopram, fluoxetine, paroxetine, and sertraline also exhibit antimuscarinic activity; dopamine reuptake is inhibited by paroxetine and sertraline; and sertraline weakly antagonizes α-adrenergic receptors.[17] Despite their relative receptor selectivity, SSRIs can be proconvulsant in the setting of an overdose.[30] How this occurs is still not known.

Overdose of SSRIs can cause serotonin syndrome. Although seizures may be more likely to occur in this setting, not all SSRI overdose–induced seizures result from serotonin syndrome.[30,31] This class of antidepressants can also cause hyponatremia brought on by the syndrome of inappropriate antidiuretic hormone secretion (SIADH)[32] and this mechanism has caused seizures with therapeutic use of paroxetine[33] and could potentially cause a seizure after SSRI overdose. Inhibition of glycine receptors could also play a role in SSRI overdose–induced seizures.[34] Special mention should be made of citalopram, which is a racemic mixture, containing both R and S enantiomers, whereas escitalopram contains the S enantiomer.[35] Some investigators have suggested that the R enantiomer of citalopram is responsible for the more serious toxic effects (QTc prolongation and seizures) of this drug,[35] whereas others have speculated that seizures induced by citalopram may occur from inhibition of GIRK channels.[13]

Atypical Antidepressants (Bupropion, Duloxetine, Mirtazapine, Reboxetine, Trazodone, Venlafaxine)

Atypical antidepressants consist of those drugs not belonging to the MAOI, SSRI, or CA classes. These drugs are new, share structural similarity with the SSRIs, and were developed with the intent of reducing the side effects associated with MAOIs and CAs. All of the agents in this class inhibit the reuptake of biogenic amines as part of their pharmacologic mechanism of action. In general, the mechanism(s) responsible for overdose-induced seizures for this class of antidepressants remains poorly understood. Duloxetine and reboxetine are not discussed because data are limited regarding overdose with these antidepressant drugs.

Bupropion

Bupropion is an antidepressant that increases the risk of seizures in a dose-related manner. In 1986, it was removed from the US market because of its seizure propensity, especially when patients took high doses.[36] Reintroduced in 1989, it was recommended that total daily doses not exceed 450 mg.[29] Currently, bupropion is indicated for the treatment of depression and used as an adjunct for smoking cessation. It is available in immediate-release (IR), sustained-release (SR), and extended-release (XL) formulations.

The pharmacology of bupropion is not well defined. Bupropion and its active metabolite, hydroxybupropion, inhibit the reuptake of dopamine and, to a lesser degree, norepinephrine and serotonin.[37] Hydroxybupropion may be the causative agent for seizures associated with high therapeutic doses of bupropion or after an overdose. Hydroxybupropion and other metabolites have been detected in much higher concentrations compared with bupropion in patients who have experienced bupropion-induced seizures and in individuals who have died of bupropion overdose.[38,39] However, the precise mechanism for hydroxybupropion-induced seizures remains to be elucidated.

Mirtazapine

Mirtazapine was first introduced for clinical use in 2001 and has a distinctive mechanism of action. It inhibits the reuptake of serotonin; antagonizes H_1 receptors; and antagonizes α_2-adrenergic receptors, which increases neuronal norepinephrine and serotonin concentrations.[40] In addition, mirtazapine blocks some serotonin receptor subtypes including 5-HT$_2$ and 5-HT$_3$.[41] The underlying mechanism for mirtazapine overdose–induced seizures is currently unknown.

Trazodone

The main pharmacologic mechanism of action of trazodone is mediated through antagonism of 5-HT$_{2A}$ receptors and inhibition of serotonin reuptake.[42] It also antagonizes peripheral α_1-adrenergic receptors and has equivocal affinity for H$_1$ histamine receptors.[24] In rare instances, trazodone can cause hyponatremia through SIADH[43] and this is one reason that may account for seizures after overdose of trazodone.[44]

Venlafaxine

The pathways responsible for seizure activity associated with venlafaxine overdose are likely multiple. This selective norepinephrine/serotonin reuptake inhibitor shares a similar structure and pharmacology to that of tramadol,[45] which has also been reported to cause seizures after overdose.[46] Serotonin toxicity[45] or sodium channel blockade[47] may account for its seizure propensity after intentional ingestion.

EXAMINING THE EVIDENCE FOR ANTIDEPRESSANT OVERDOSE–INDUCED SEIZURES

Before examining the evidence for antidepressant overdose–induced seizures, it is important to recognize the various sources of available clinical data. First and foremost, there are no randomized controlled trials that have evaluated this problem. Much of our knowledge and understanding of antidepressant overdose–induced seizures is based on case reports, case series, observational studies, and retrospective analyses. These methodologies have obvious inherent limitations, and the clinical evidence for antidepressant overdose–induced seizures in many instances may also be hindered by (1) the lack of any control for predisposing risk factors, (2) failure to account for the presence of an underlying seizure disorder, (3) absence of serum drug concentrations, (4) inaccurate reporting of drug doses ingested, or (5) difficulty in determining whether the seizure was caused by the antidepressant or another factor such as a coingestant or a cardiovascular phenomenon that produced a decrease in cerebral perfusion. Nevertheless, these methodologies currently provide the best available evidence with which to evaluate antidepressant overdose–induced seizures in human subjects. **Table 1** provides a quick reference tool that risk stratifies antidepressants for their seizure propensity in overdose.

MAOIS

Reflective of their dwindling use in the clinical arena, human exposures to MAOIs reported to the NPDS in 2009 accounted for only 0.23% (n = 234) of all antidepressant exposures.[2] Seizures after an overdose of a MAOI and with therapeutic use are rare, with few cases reported.[48,49] A subgroup analysis of single-substance overdoses of phenelzine and tranylcypromine reported in a 5-year period found that 2 out of 56 patients who had ingested phenelzine experienced seizure activity, whereas 1 out of 35 patients who had ingested tranylcypromine developed seizure activity.[50] The preponderance of evidence suggests that MAOI overdose–induced seizures typically happen in the setting of polysubstance ingestion or with the development of serotonin syndrome.[51,52] Further supporting this notion is a report that analyzed 106 moclobemide overdose cases.[53] No seizures occurred with the sole ingestion of moclobemide, whereas the concomitant overdose of moclobemide and serotonergic coingestants

Table 1
Risk stratification for antidepressant overdose–induced seizures[a]

Antidepressant Class Representative Drugs from Each Class	Risk for Antidepressant Overdose–induced Seizures		
	Low Risk <5% Seizure Incidence After Overdose	Intermediate Risk 5%–10% Seizure Incidence After Overdose	High Risk >10% Seizure Incidence After Overdose
MAOIs			
Isocarboxazid[b]	+	−	−
Moclobemide	+	−	−
Phenelzine[b]	+	−	−
Selegiline[b]	+	−	−
Tranylcypromine[b]	+	−	−
CAs			
Tertiary amines			
Amitriptyline	−	+	−
Clomipramine	−	+	−
Doxepin	−	+	−
Imipramine	−	−	+
Trimipramine	−	+	−
Secondary Amines			
Desipramine	−	−	+
Nortriptyline	−	−	+
Protriptyline	−	+	−
Other			
Amoxapine	−	−	+
Maprotiline	−	−	+
SSRIs			
Citalopram[c]	−	+	−
Escitalopram	+	−	−
Fluoxetine	+	−	−
Fluvoxamine	+	−	−
Paroxetine	+	−	−
Sertraline	+	−	−
Atypical Antidepressants			
Bupropion	−	−	+
Duloxetine	Risk unknown	−	−
Mirtazapine	+	−	−
Reboxetine	Risk unknown	−	−
Trazodone	+	−	−
Venlafaxine[d]	−	+	−

[a] Data compiled from multiple sources referenced throughout the article. The table was constructed solely by the authors.
[b] Seizure risk with overdose presumed to be low based on lack of convincing clinical evidence and/or the drug shares a similar structure and/or pharmacologic mechanism to drugs within its class that have been determined to be low risk.
[c] Seizure risk with overdose should be considered high with ingestions exceeding 600 mg.
[d] Seizure risk may be high with large ingestions.

increased the risk for serotonin syndrome and seizures. Therefore, based on the rarity with which deliberate single-agent ingestions of MAOIs cause seizures, this class of antidepressants should be considered low risk for triggering a seizure after overdose.

CAS

Seizures from CA overdose were reported shortly after the introduction of imipramine in the late 1950s.[54] Since then, a sizeable body of evidence has been published substantiating the propensity for this class of antidepressants to cause seizures in overdose.

Most CA overdose–induced seizures occur within 1 to 2 hours after ingestion and typically are generalized and brief.[55] Status epilepticus with CA poisoning can develop but is unusual. However, seizures from CA poisoning are associated with an increase in mortality,[23] and patients can experience cardiovascular collapse within moments of seizing or while they are seizing.[56] This sudden deterioration is probably caused by enhanced cardiac sodium ion channel blockade that results from the development of a seizure-induced metabolic acidosis.

Several clinical markers have been investigated to predict the risk for developing seizures after CA overdose, including level of consciousness,[57] CA serum concentrations, and QRS duration on the electrocardiogram (ECG).[58] The usefulness of serum CA concentrations after overdose is limited by the difficulty in rapid determination of quantitative CA concentrations and the lack of correlation between life-threatening toxicity and drug concentrations; however, CA serum concentrations greater than 1000 ng/mL are typically linked with significant toxicity.[59] The ECG may aid in predicting which patients are at risk for seizures after CA overdose. For example, one study found that 34% of patients with a QRS duration greater than or equal to 100 milliseconds experienced seizures, whereas no seizures occurred in patients with QRS durations less than 100 milliseconds.[58] Additional studies have shown that a QRS duration greater than 100 milliseconds is associated with serious CA toxicity such as dysrhythmias and seizures.[60,61] However, a normal ECG or QRS duration less than 100 milliseconds cannot be used to exclude the possible development of seizures or other complications after CA overdose.[62,63] A meta-analysis found a pooled sensitivity of 0.69 and specificity of 0.69 for predicting seizures using QRS duration.[64] Comprehensive discussion of prognostic indicators after CA overdose is beyond the scope of this article, and the reader is referred elsewhere for further information.[64]

The incidence of seizures with CA toxicity is varied, ranging from 3% to more than 20%.[65–67] A review that compiled data on 2536 patients from 26 studies of CA overdose reported an overall incidence of 8.4% for CA overdose–induced seizures.[23] An analysis of single-agent suicidal antidepressant ingestions reported to US poison centers from 2000 to 2004 listed the incidence of overdose-induced seizure activity for individual CAs in order of increasing percentage: protriptyline (0%), trimipramine (0%), amitriptyline (3.5%), nortriptyline (4.8%), doxepin (5.2%), clomipramine (6.9%), imipramine (10.5%), and desipramine (14.5%).[50] Other studies with overdose of individual CAs have revealed a high rate of seizures with desipramine (17.9%), imipramine (20.6%), and nortriptyline (22.2%).[65,66] Tabulating the true incidence of seizures for specific CAs is challenging because several of the CAs are infrequently involved in overdose (eg, protriptyline, and trimipramine).[2,50] Based on current knowledge, patients should be stratified as high risk for seizures after toxic ingestions of desipramine, imipramine, and nortriptyline, and intermediate risk for seizures after toxic ingestions of amitriptyline, clomipramine, doxepin, protriptyline, and trimipramine.

Amoxapine

In acute overdose, amoxapine is troublesome. Among 33 patients who overdosed on amoxapine, seizure activity occurred in 36.4% compared with 4.3% in other CA poisonings.[25] This study also showed that the mortality with amoxapine overdose was almost 22 times greater compared with overdose of all other CAs. A study of human exposures to antidepressants reported to the Maryland Poison Control Center in a 2-year period found that 21.7% of patients who had ingested amoxapine alone experienced seizure activity.[65] Moreover, a recent analysis of poison control data found that 29.2% of patients experienced seizure activity after isolated amoxapine ingestions.[50] Because amoxapine overdose has a high likelihood of causing seizures, and because these seizures can be difficult to control,[25] or deteriorate to status epilepticus,[68] this antidepressant should be deemed high risk for causing seizures after overdose.

Maprotiline

There is a significant risk for seizures from maprotiline in acute overdose. A study comparing the relative cardiac and CNS toxicity of amoxapine, maprotiline, and trazodone with older CAs found that 18% of patients developed a seizure after isolated maprotiline overdose.[65] In addition, although only 19 cases of isolated maprotiline ingestions were reported to US poison centers from 2000 to 2004, almost 16% of patients experienced seizure activity.[50] Despite the infrequent use of maprotiline today, it should be labeled high risk for inducing seizure activity after an overdose.

SSRIS

Although this class of antidepressants is believed to be generally safe in overdose, all SSRIs can cause overdose-induced seizures.[30,34] The seizure risk from escitalopram, fluoxetine, fluvoxamine, paroxetine, and sertraline overdose is low. A prospective multicenter study that analyzed 87 cases of isolated fluoxetine ingestion reported no seizures.[69] In a cohort study of 233 first admissions of deliberate self-poisoning with a single SSRI, seizures occurred in only 1.3% of patients.[45] A retrospective cohort study that compared the clinical features of deliberate self-poisoning with venlafaxine and SSRIs reported a seizure rate of 2.3% after SSRI overdose.[70] A review of SSRI poisoning admissions to an Australian toxicology unit reported a seizure incidence of 2% for citalopram, 1% for fluoxetine, 4% for fluvoxamine, 2% for paroxetine, and 2% for sertraline.[30]

Several retrospective reviews evaluating monointoxication with either citalopram or escitalopram have revealed that citalopram has a greater tendency for causing seizures after overdose. First, Ho and colleagues[71] found that seizures occurred in 7.5% of patients who ingested citalopram (median dose 536 mg) alone compared with 3% of patients who ingested escitalopram (median dose 222 mg) alone. Second, Hayes and colleagues[35] evaluated single-substance acute overdoses with citalopram and escitalopram; seizures were described more commonly with citalopram (8%) than with escitalopram (0.2%). Third, isolated citalopram and escitalopram overdoses reported to several European poison centers from 1997 to 2006 were retrospectively analyzed; seizures occurred in 13.6% of cases after citalopram overdose compared with 1.6% after escitalopram overdose.[34] When seizures occur after citalopram overdose, they are typically generalized, self-limited, or terminate with benzodiazepines, and develop within 1 to 13 hours after ingestion.[72]

The risk of citalopram overdose–induced seizures escalates in a dose-related fashion. Waring and colleagues[72] found that, in the absence of coingestants, the minimum dose of citalopram associated with seizures was 400 mg. Hayes and colleagues[35] reported a 3% incidence of seizures in patients ingesting less than 600 mg citalopram, 11.6% seizure incidence for ingestions between 600 and 1900 mg, and 75% incidence of seizures for ingestions greater than 1900 mg. A study by Yilmaz and colleagues[34] showed seizures in 11% of cases at doses of 400 to 800 mg citalopram; 27% of cases at doses of 802 to 1200 mg; 41% of cases at doses of 1202 to 1600 mg; and 52% of cases at doses greater than 1600 mg. Clinical evidence for citalopram overdose–induced seizures continues to mount. Although it is difficult to determine an exact dose at which seizures will occur with citalopram overdose, current data suggest that this antidepressant should be categorized as intermediate risk with ingestions between 400 and 600 mg, and high risk when doses exceed 600 mg.

ATYPICAL ANTIDEPRESSANTS
Bupropion

Several studies have shown that the IR, SR, and XL formulations of bupropion have a high incidence of seizures in overdose.[73–75] Seizure activity occurred in 21% of patients with overdose involving the IR formulation,[73] 11% of patients who primarily overdosed on the SR formulation,[74] and 32% of patients who overdosed on the XL formulation.[75] Seizures induced by overdose of bupropion are problematic because they can be multiple[50] and can progress to status epilepticus.[5] As an example, analysis of US poison control data from 2000 to 2004 revealed 7631 cases of solitary bupropion ingestions; 801 cases involved a single seizure, 450 cases involved multiple seizures, and 61 cases involved status epilepticus.[50] Furthermore, Starr and colleagues[75] reported that almost one-half of the patients in their observational study of bupropion XL overdoses had experienced more than 1 seizure.

Another problem with bupropion overdose–induced seizures is the delayed onset with which they can occur. Seizure activity has been reported to occur up to 8 hours (mean, 3.7 hours),[73] 14 hours (mean, 4.3 hours),[74] and 24 hours (mean, 7.3 hours)[75] after overdose on the IR, SR, and XL preparations, respectively. Even though patients who develop a bupropion overdose–induced seizure are more likely to have agitation or tremor on physical examination before seizing, these seizures can develop in patients lacking any signs or symptoms of CNS toxicity.[75] Based on the high incidence of seizures after overdose of bupropion, and because these seizures can be multiple or delayed in their onset, this drug should be labeled as high risk after overdose.

Mirtazapine

Not much is known about mirtazapine overdose and data continue to accumulate. A retrospective chart review of mirtazapine ingestions reported to a US poison center in 2004 identified 33 intentional and isolated mirtazapine ingestions; no seizures were reported to have occurred.[41] Mirtazapine accounted for 3.1% (n = 2599) of single-agent suicidal antidepressant ingestions reported to US poison centers from 2000 to 2004 and a single seizure occurred in 5 cases.[50] A retrospective analysis reported no seizure activity with 117 cases of mirtazapine overdose admitted to a Scottish toxicology unit during a 5-year period.[40] However, the investigators of the same study postulated that, given the study size, a power of 87% to detect a 3% risk of seizures, and assuming a background frequency of 0.1%, that the true risk of seizures with mirtazapine overdose could be as high as 2.6%. Existing evidence supports that this antidepressant is low risk for overdose-induced seizures.

Trazodone

With the exception of CNS depression and mild hypotension, the effects of trazodone when ingested as a single agent in deliberate self-poisonings are not severe.[76]

Seizures have been reported after trazodone overdose but are uncommon.[77] Between the years 2000 and 2004, trazodone accounted for 15.1% (n = 12,538) of single-agent suicidal antidepressant ingestions reported to US poison centers, and a single seizure occurred in 13 cases.[50] Because seizures have been shown to occur only sporadically after the intentional ingestion of trazodone as a sole agent, this atypical antidepressant should be categorized as low risk for overdose-induced seizures.

Venlafaxine

Venlafaxine was previously considered to have low toxicity with overdose compared with MAOIs and CAs.[17] However, newer evidence from a comparison of fatality indices suggests that venlafaxine is more toxic than SSRIs and at least as toxic as clomipramine and nortriptyline.[78] Venlafaxine has shown a greater proclivity toward seizures with overdose compared with drugs within some of the other antidepressant classes. In a 2003 prospective cohort study, seizures occurred in approximately 14% of venlafaxine overdoses and were more frequent than SSRI and tricyclic antidepressant overdose–induced seizures.[45] All of the patients who had experienced a venlafaxine overdose–induced seizure had ingested 900 mg or more. In a comparative analysis performed by White and colleagues,[50] venlafaxine caused seizure activity in 220 out of 5510 patients ($\sim$4%) who had ingested it in a suicidal overdose; 11 of the patients were reported to have experienced status epilepticus. Recently, a retrospective cohort study assessed 36 patients with venlafaxine self-poisoning and 44 randomly selected patients with SSRI self-poisoning; seizures were recorded in 8.3% of the venlafaxine cases compared with 2.3% of the SSRI cases.[70] Because there is an evolving body of evidence that continues to reveal the proconvulsant effects of venlafaxine with overdose, it should be ranked as intermediate risk for overdose-induced seizures; however, large ingestions may increase this risk.

TREATMENT CONSIDERATIONS

Evaluating and treating a patient who has overdosed on an antidepressant can pose several challenges to the clinician.

1. Patients may present with altered mental status, significantly limiting the ability to take an adequate history.
2. The patient may have ingested other substances contributing to their clinical presentation.
3. Some antidepressants, such as bupropion and citalopram, can cause delayed-onset seizures.
4. Antidepressant overdose–induced seizures can deteriorate to status epilepticus.
5. In addition to causing neurotoxicity, several antidepressants can result in life-threatening cardiotoxicity that requires prompt antidotal therapy.

After assessing the patient's airway and vital signs, a focused history should be obtained and a physical examination performed. The exposure history can be supported by findings on the physical examination such as agitation, CNS depression, diaphoresis, mydriasis, or tachycardia. The patient may have a specific toxidrome after ingestion of an antidepressant (eg, anticholinergic from CA overdose, serotonin syndrome from SSRI overdose, or sympathomimetic from MAOI or venlafaxine overdose). Intravenous access should be established, and the patient placed on a cardiac monitor and under seizure precautions. Although the benefits of gastrointestinal decontamination are controversial,[79] activated charcoal at a dose of 1 g/kg should be considered when an ingestion of an antidepressant is potentially life-threatening, or an SR formulation was ingested. To decrease the likelihood of aspiration, awake patients should be able to protect their airway or, if a patient is intubated, the airway should be secured with a cuffed endotracheal tube before administration of activated charcoal.

Because many poisoned patients are unable or unwilling to provide a reliable history, laboratory evaluation is crucial. Rapid determination of blood glucose should be performed for all patients with altered mental status or those who are actively seizing. Diagnostic tests, such as a comprehensive metabolic panel and ECG, provide invaluable information regarding end-organ toxicity and insight into potential deterioration in a patient's condition. A quantitative test for common coingestants, for instance acetaminophen or aspirin, may be warranted, whereas quantitative testing of specific antidepressants is not recommended. The routine use of serum and urine drug screens in the acute overdose patient is infrequently beneficial.

Risk factors for seizures should be identified and include history of seizures, head trauma, polypharmacy, CNS lesions, and concomitant substance abuse or withdrawal.[27] **Table 1** can be used to help determine the risk of seizures after overdose of various antidepressants. If the patient is actively seizing, benzodiazepines such as diazepam, lorazepam, or midazolam are considered first-line therapy. Second-line therapy includes phenobarbital. If large doses of these agents are used, or if the patient develops refractory seizures, then intubation may be necessary for airway protection and ventilation. If neuromuscular blockade is necessary to facilitate intubation, then a nondepolarizing agent with a short duration of action, like rocuronium, should be used.[80] The use of long-acting paralytics should be avoided; however, if a drug such as pancuronium has to be used, then bedside electroencephalographic monitoring should be instituted.

If seizures are refractory to benzodiazepine and barbiturate therapy, propofol has been used successfully used to treat antidepressant overdose-induced seizures.[68] Patients who develop refractory seizures from ingestions of a hydrazine derivate, or when the ingestion is unknown, should be treated with pyridoxine. Phenytoin, although second-line therapy for most seizures, is usually not effective for the treatment of drug-induced seizures or CA overdose–induced seizures.[6,81] Patients who are seizing from an antidepressant that causes cardiac sodium channel blockade should be treated simultaneously with 1 to 2 mEq/kg of sodium bicarbonate given as an intravenous bolus in addition to conventional therapy and repeated as needed until a blood pH of 7.55 is attained[82,83]; sodium bicarbonate is effective for treating drug-induced cardiac sodium channel blockade.[84] In addition, lipid emulsion, a novel therapy believed to work by pulling lipid-soluble drugs out of tissues, has been used to successfully restore circulation in a patient who experienced seizure activity and cardiovascular collapse after overdose of bupropion and lamotrigine.[85]

The process of determining disposition after an antidepressant overdose is not always straightforward. Any patient who has overdosed on an antidepressant and is displaying signs or symptoms of toxicity should be admitted for further evaluation and treatment. In many instances, patients can be observed for a period of 4 to 6 hours after ingestion. If they remain without signs or symptoms of toxicity, a decision on disposition can be rendered; the patient may require psychiatric evaluation or can be discharged home. Patients who have ingested CAs and who are asymptomatic on presentation, receive activated charcoal, remain asymptomatic for a minimum of 6 hours in the treating facility without any treatment intervention, and have normal ECGs can receive disposition as deemed appropriate.[86] Some exceptions that necessitate prolonged monitoring include ingestion of (1) sustained-release formulations, (2) drugs that can cause delayed-onset seizures (eg, bupropion or citalopram), or (3) antidepressants that can cause cardiotoxicity, such as bupropion,[85] citalopram and escitalopram,[35] or venlafaxine.[45]

SUMMARY

Deliberate self-ingestion of antidepressants is a problem commonly encountered in emergency departments throughout the United States. Because seizures are a serious complication of antidepressant overdose, clinicians should recognize the risk associated with overdose of various antidepressants. Understanding the seizure potential of antidepressants in overdose can help to determine the need for inpatient monitoring and assist in treatment decisions for clinicians.

REFERENCES

1. Olfson M, Marcus SC. National patterns in antidepressant medication treatment. Arch Gen Psychiatry 2009;66:848–56.
2. Bronstein AC, Spyker DA, Cantilena LR Jr, et al. 2009 annual report of the American Association of Poison Control Centers' National Poison Data System (NPDS): 27th Annual Report. Clin Toxicol 2010;48:979–1178.
3. Beuhler MC, Spiller HA, Sasser HC. The outcome of unintentional pediatric bupropion ingestions: a NPDS database review. J Med Toxicol 2010;6:4–8.
4. Pisani F, Oteri G, Costa C, et al. Effects of psychotropic drugs on seizure threshold. Drug Saf 2002;25:91–110.
5. Thundiyil JG, Kearney TE, Olson KR. Evolving epidemiology of drug-induced seizures reported to a poison control center system. J Med Toxicol 2007;3:15–9.
6. Wills B, Erickson T. Chemically induced seizures. Clin Lab Med 2006;26:185–209.
7. Clark M, Post RM. Carbamazepine, but not caffeine, is highly selective for adenosine A_1 binding sites. Eur J Pharmacol 1989;164:399–401.
8. Malatynska E, Knapp RJ, Ikeda M, et al. Antidepressants and seizure-interactions at the GABA-receptor chloride-ionophore complex. Life Sci 1988;43:303–7.
9. Yokoyama H, Iinuma K. Histamine and seizures: implications for the treatment of epilepsy. CNS Drugs 1996;5:321–30.
10. Tuovinen K. Organophosphate-induced convulsions and prevention of neuropathological damages. Toxicology 2004;196:31–9.
11. Teitelbaum JS, Zatorre RJ, Carpenter S, et al. Neurologic sequelae of domoic acid intoxication due to the ingestion of contaminated mussels. N Engl J Med 1990;322:1781–7.
12. DeToledo JC. Lidocaine and seizures. Ther Drug Monit 2000;22:320–2.
13. Jobe PC, Browning RA. The serotonergic and noradrenergic effects of antidepressant drugs are anticonvulsant, not proconvulsant. Epilepsy Behav 2005;7: 602–19.
14. Dailey JW, Naritoku DK. Antidepressants and seizures: clinical anecdotes overshadow neuroscience. Biochem Pharmacol 1996;52:1323–9.
15. Krishnan KR. Revisiting monoamine oxidase inhibitors. J Clin Psychiatry 2007; 68(Suppl 8):35–41.
16. Bonnet U. Moclobemide: evolution, pharmacodynamic, and pharmacokinetic properties. CNS Drug Rev 2002;8:283–308.
17. Richelson E. Pharmacology of antidepressants. Mayo Clin Proc 2001;76:511–27.
18. Frieling H, Bleich S. Tranylcypromine: new perspectives on an "old" drug. Eur Arch Psychiatry Clin Neurosci 2006;256:268–73.
19. Bonnet U. Moclobemide: therapeutic use and clinical studies. CNS Drug Rev 2003;9:97–140.

20. Judge BS. Differentiating the causes of metabolic acidosis in the poisoned patient. Clin Lab Med 2006;26:31–48.
21. Squires RF, Saederup H. Antidepressants and metabolites that block GABA$_A$ receptors coupled to ^{35}S-t-butylbicyclophosphorothionate binding sites in rat brain. Brain Res 1988;441:15–22.
22. Shioda K, Nisijima K, Yoshino T, et al. Extracellular serotonin, dopamine and glutamate levels are elevated in the hypothalamus in a serotonin syndrome animal model induced by tranylcypromine and fluoxetine. Prog Neuropsychopharmacol Biol Psychiatry 2004;28:633–40.
23. Frommer DA, Kulig KW, Marx JA, et al. Tricyclic antidepressant overdose. JAMA 1987;257:521–6.
24. Rudorfer MV, Manji HK, Potter WZ. Comparative tolerability profiles of the newer versus older antidepressants. Drug Saf 1994;10:18–46.
25. Litovitz TL, Troutman WG. Amoxapine overdose: seizures and fatalities. JAMA 1983;250:1069–71.
26. Kumlien E, Lundberg PO. Seizure risk associated with neuroactive drugs: Data from the WHO adverse drug reactions database. Seizure 2010;19:69–73.
27. Skowron DM, Stimmel GL. Antidepressants and the risk of seizures. Pharmacotherapy 1992;12:18–22.
28. Jabbari B, Bryan GE, March EE, et al. Incidence of seizures with tricyclic and tetracyclic antidepressants. Arch Neurol 1985;42:480–1.
29. Lee KC, Finley PR, Alldredge BK. Risk of seizures associated with psychotropic medications: emphasis on new drugs and new findings. Expert Opin Drug Saf 2003;2:233–47.
30. Isbister GK, Bowe SJ, Dawson A, et al. Relative toxicity of selective serotonin reuptake inhibitors (SSRIs) in overdose. J Toxicol Clin Toxicol 2004;42:277–85.
31. Suchard JR. Fluoxetine overdose-induced seizure. West J Emerg Med 2008;9: 154–6.
32. Kirchner V, Silver LE, Kelly CA. Selective serotonin reuptake inhibitors and hyponatraemia: review and proposed mechanisms in the elderly. J Psychopharmacol 1998;12:396–400.
33. Corrington KA, Gatlin CC, Fields KB. A case of SSRI-induced hyponatremia. J Am Board Fam Pract 2002;15:63–5.
34. Yilmaz Z, Ceschi A, Rauber-Lüthy C, et al. Escitalopram causes fewer seizures in human overdose than citalopram. Clin Toxicol 2010;48:207–12.
35. Hayes BD, Klein-Schwartz W, Clark RF, et al. Comparison of toxicity of acute overdoses with citalopram and escitalopram. J Emerg Med 2010;39:44–8.
36. Alldredge BK. Seizure risk associated with psychotropic drugs: clinical and pharmacokinetic considerations. Neurology 1999;53(Suppl 2):S68–75.
37. Ascher JA, Cole JO, Colin JN, et al. Bupropion: a review of its mechanism of antidepressant activity. J Clin Psychiatry 1995;56:395–401.
38. Friel PN, Logan BK, Fligner CL. Three fatal drug overdoses involving bupropion. J Anal Toxicol 1993;17:436–8.
39. Davidson J. Seizures and bupropion: a review. J Clin Psychiatry 1989;50:256–61.
40. Waring WS, Good AM, Bateman DN. Lack of significant toxicity after mirtazapine overdose: a five-year review of cases admitted to a regional toxicology unit. Clin Toxicol 2007;45:45–50.
41. LoVecchio F, Riley B, Pizon A, et al. Outcomes after isolated mirtazapine (Remeron) supratherapeutic ingestions. J Emerg Med 2008;34:77–8.
42. Montgomery SA. Antidepressants and seizures: emphasis on newer agents and clinical implications. Int J Clin Pract 2005;59:1435–40.

43. Spigset O, Hedenmalm K. Hyponatraemia and the syndrome of inappropriate antidiuretic hormone secretion (SIADH) induced by psychotropic drugs. Drug Saf 1995;12:209–25.

44. Vanpee D, Laloyaux P, Gillet JB. Seizure and hyponatremia after overdose of trazodone. Am J Emerg Med 1999;17:430–1.

45. Whyte IM, Dawson AH, Buckley NA. Relative toxicity of venlafaxine and selective serotonin reuptake inhibitors in overdose compared to tricyclic antidepressants. QJM 2003;96:369–74.

46. Tobias J. Seizure after overdose of tramadol. South Med J 1997;90:826–7.

47. Khalifa M, Daleau P, Turgeon J. Mechanism of sodium channel block by venlafaxine in guinea pig ventricular myocytes. J Pharmacol Exp Ther 1999;291:280–4.

48. Bhugra DK, Kaye N. Phenelizine induced grand mal seizure. Br J Clin Pract 1986; 40:173–4.

49. Albareda M, Udina C, Escartín A, et al. Seizures in a diabetic patient on monoamine oxidase inhibitors. Am J Emerg Med 1999;17:107–8.

50. White NC, Litovitz T, Clancy C. Suicidal antidepressant overdoses: a comparative analysis by antidepressant type. J Med Toxicol 2008;4:238–50.

51. Vouri E, Henry JA, Ojanperä I, et al. Death following ingestion of MDMA (ecstasy) and moclobemide. Addiction 2003;98:365–8.

52. Singer PP, Jones GR. An uncommon fatality due to moclobemide. J Anal Toxicol 1997;21:518–20.

53. Isbister GK, Hackett LP, Dawson AH, et al. Moclobemide poisoning: toxicokinetics and occurrence of serotonin toxicity. Br J Clin Pharmacol 2003;56:441–50.

54. Zaccara G, Muscas GC, Messori A. Clinical features, pathogenesis and management of drug-induced seizures. Drug Saf 1990;5:109–51.

55. Ellison DW, Pentel PR. Clinical features and consequences of seizures due to cyclic antidepressant overdose. Am J Emerg Med 1989;7:5–10.

56. Taboulet P, Michard R, Muszynski J, et al. Cardiovascular repercussions of seizures during cyclic antidepressant poisoning. J Toxicol Clin Toxicol 1995;33: 205–11.

57. Hultén BÅ, Adams R, Askenasi R, et al. Predicting severity of tricyclic antidepressant overdose. J Toxicol Clin Toxicol 1992;30:161–70.

58. Boehnert MT, Lovejoy FH Jr. Value of the QRS duration versus the serum drug level in predicting seizures and ventricular arrhythmias after an acute overdose of tricyclic antidepressants. N Engl J Med 1985;313:474–9.

59. Lavoie FW, Gansert GG, Weiss RE. Value of initial ECG findings and plasma drug levels in cyclic antidepressant overdose. Ann Emerg Med 1990;19:696–700.

60. Caravati EM, Bossart PJ. Demographic and electrocardiographic factors associated with severe tricyclic antidepressant toxicity. J Toxicol Clin Toxicol 1991;29: 31–43.

61. Leibelt EL, Francis PD, Woolf AD. ECG lead aVR versus QRS interval in predicting seizures and arrhythmias in acute tricyclic antidepressant toxicity. Ann Emerg Med 1995;26:195–201.

62. Buckley NA, Dawson AH. Greater toxicity in overdose of dothiepin than of other tricyclic antidepressants. Lancet 1994;343:159–62.

63. Foulke GE, Albertson TE. QRS interval in tricyclic antidepressant overdosage: inaccuracy as a toxicity indicator in emergency settings. Ann Emerg Med 1987; 16:160–3.

64. Bailey B, Buckley NA, Amre DK. A meta-analysis of prognostic indicators to predict seizures, arrhythmias, or death after tricyclic antidepressant overdose. J Toxicol Clin Toxicol 2004;42:877–88.

65. Wedin GP, Oderda GM, Klein-Schwartz W. Relative toxicity of cyclic antidepressants. Ann Emerg Med 1986;15:797–804.
66. Crome P, Newman B. The problem of tricyclic antidepressant poisoning. Postgrad Med J 1979;55:528–32.
67. Strøm J, Madsen PS, Nielsen NN, et al. Acute self-poisoning with tricyclic antidepressants in 295 consecutive patients treated in an ICU. Acta Anaesthesiol Scand 1984;28:666–70.
68. Merigian KS, Browning RG, Leeper KV. Successful treatment of amoxapine-induced refractory status epilepticus with propofol (Diprivan). Acad Emerg Med 1995;2:128–33.
69. Borys DJ, Setzer SC, Ling LJ, et al. Acute fluoxetine overdose: a report of 234 cases. Am J Emerg Med 1992;10:115–20.
70. Chan AN, Gunja N, Ryan CJ. A comparison of venlafaxine and SSRIs in deliberate self-poisoning. J Med Toxicol 2010;6:116–21.
71. Ho R, Norman RF, van Veen MM, et al. A 3-year review of citalopram and escitalopram ingestions [abstract]. J Toxicol Clin Toxicol 2004;42:746.
72. Waring WS, Gray JA, Graham A. Predictive factors for generalized seizures after deliberate citalopram overdose. Br J Clin Pharmacol 2008;66:861–5.
73. Spiller HA, Ramoska EA, Sheen SR, et al. Bupropion overdose: a 3-year multicenter retrospective analysis. Am J Emerg Med 1994;12:43–5.
74. Shepherd G, Velez LI, Keyes DC. Intentional bupropion overdoses. J Emerg Med 2004;27:147–51.
75. Starr P, Klein-Schwartz W, Spiller H, et al. Incidence and onset of delayed seizures after overdoses of extended-release bupropion. Am J Emerg Med 2009;27:911–5.
76. Sarko J. Antidepressants, old and new: a review of their adverse effects and toxicity in overdose. Emerg Med Clin North Am 2000;18:637–54.
77. Gamble DE. Trazodone overdose: four years of experience from voluntary reports. J Clin Psychiatry 1986;47:544–6.
78. Buckley NA, McManus PR. Fatal toxicity of serotoninergic and other antidepressant drugs: analysis of United Kingdom mortality data. BMJ 2002;325:1332–3.
79. Heard K. The changing indications of gastrointestinal decontamination. Clin Lab Med 2006;26:1–12.
80. Marik PE, Varon J. The management of status epilepticus. Chest 2004;126:582–91.
81. Pimentel L, Trommer L. Cyclic antidepressant overdoses: a review. Emerg Med Clin North Am 1994;12:533–47.
82. Smilkstein MJ. Reviewing cyclic antidepressant cardiotoxicity: wheat and chaff. J Emerg Med 1990;8:645–8.
83. Pentel PR, Benowitz NL. Tricyclic antidepressant poisoning. Management of arrhythmias. Med Toxicol 1986;1:101–21.
84. Hoffman JR, Votey SR, Bayer M, et al. Effect of hypertonic sodium bicarbonate in the treatment of moderate-to-severe cyclic antidepressant overdose. Am J Emerg Med 1993;11:336–41.
85. Sirianni AJ, Osterhoudt KC, Calello DP, et al. Use of lipid emulsion in the resuscitation of a patient with prolonged cardiovascular collapse after overdose of bupropion and lamotrigine. Ann Emerg Med 2008;51:412–5.
86. Banahan BF Jr, Schelkun PH. Tricyclic antidepressant overdose: conservative management in a community hospital with cost-saving implications. J Emerg Med 1990;8:451–4.

Neurologic Manifestations of Chronic Methamphetamine Abuse

Daniel E. Rusyniak, MD

KEYWORDS

- Methamphetamine abuse • Psychosis • Parkinson's • Choreoathetoid • Punding
- Formication

COMMENTARY ON METHAMPHETAMINE ABUSE FOR PSYCHIATRIC PRACTICE

Every decade seems to have its own unique drug problem. The 1970s had hallucinogens, the 1980s had crack cocaine, the 1990s had designer drugs, the 2000s had methamphetamine (Meth), and in the 2010s we are dealing with the scourge of prescription drug abuse. While each of these drug epidemics has distinctive problems and history, the one with perhaps the greatest impact on the practice of Psychiatry is Meth. By increasing the extracellular concentrations of dopamine while slowly damaging the dopaminergic neurotransmission, Meth is a powerfully addictive drug whose chronic use preferentially causes psychiatric complications. Chronic Meth users have deficits in memory and executive functioning as well as higher rates of anxiety, depression, and most notably psychosis. It is because of addiction and chronic psychosis from Meth abuse that the Meth user is most likely to come to the attention of the practicing Psychiatrist/Psychologist.

Understanding the chronic neurologic manifestations of Meth abuse will better arm practitioners with the diagnostic and therapeutic tools needed to make the Meth epidemic one of historical interest only.

This article originally appeared in the *August 2011 issue of Neurologic Clinics (Volume 29, Number 3)*.

This work was supported by USPHS grants DA020484 and DA026867.

The author has nothing to disclose.

Department of Emergency Medicine, Indiana University School of Medicine, 1050 Wishard Boulevard, Room 2200, Indianapolis, IN 46202, USA

E-mail address: drusynia@iupui.edu

Psychiatr Clin N Am 36 (2013) 261–275

http://dx.doi.org/10.1016/j.psc.2013.02.005

0193-953X/13/$ – see front matter © 2013 Elsevier Inc. All rights reserved.

KEY POINTS

- Methamphetamine abuse can cause a chronic psychosis similar to schizophrenia.
- A common manifestation of Meth psychosis is delusional parasitosis.
- Repetitive non-goal directed behaviors (punding) can result from chronic Meth abuse.
- As with other stimulants, Meth abuse can cause choreoathetoid movements.
- Dopamine receptor antagonists are the most effective treatments for Meth's chronic psychiatric manifestations.

The current epidemic of methamphetamine abuse in the United States is not surprising. Methamphetamine can be produced from a wide variety of starting materials and methods. This fact is in contrast to cocaine, which is only commercially grown in South America, must be extracted from the plant, converted to its free-base form, shipped overseas (escaping detection by the Drug Enforcement Administration [DEA]), and then distributed, typically through gangs, to clients on the street.[1] Based on the attractiveness of methamphetamine to both users and its manufacturers, it is only surprising that the current outbreak of methamphetamine abuse in the United States took so long to reach epidemic proportions.

In 1893, methamphetamine was synthesized from ephedrine (derived from the plant *Ephedra sinica*) by Nagai Nagayoshi.[2,3] Eventually, a synthetic version would find its way to the consumer market as an over-the-counter (OTC) nasal decongestant and a brochodilator.[4–6] Far from an OTC drug today, the Food and Drug Administration (FDA) has characterized methamphetamine as a schedule II drug, which can only be prescribed for attention-deficit/hyperactivity disorder, extreme obesity, or to treat narcolepsy.

With the world on the brink of war, and its toxic effects not yet well described, the clinical effects of methamphetamine were thought to be ideal for the soldier in combat: increased alertness and aggression, plus decreased hunger and need to sleep. In World War II, the United States, Germany, and Japan all readily employed it with their troops[5,7]; it has been estimated that the United States alone distributed 200 million tablets to troops.[4] After the war, Japan experienced widespread abuse as army surpluses flooded the market. Although methamphetamine usage in Japan declined in the 1960s, it resurged in the 1970s and continues to be a problem today.[7,8] In 1954, at the height of its first epidemic, there were an estimated 2 million methamphetamine users in Japan. Although still highest in Asia, methamphetamine abuse has become a worldwide epidemic. A 2008 United Nations Office on Drugs and Crime Reports estimated 25 million abusers of amphetamines worldwide, exceeding the number of users for both cocaine (14 million) and heroin (11 million).[9]

After World War II, many US soldiers and civilians continued to use methamphetamine, which at that time was available by prescription in an injectable form. When Abbott and Burroughs-Wellcome withdrew their injectable formulations in the early 1960s, an opportunity arose for the illegal manufacturing and distribution of methamphetamine.[4] West Coast motorcycle gangs, such as the infamous Hells Angels, quickly seized on this opportunity, and by the 1970s gangs were largely responsible for the manufacturing, distribution, and use of methamphetamine in the United States. It was from the transportation of methamphetamine in the crankshafts of motorcycles that it got its street name of crank.[10] At that time, methamphetamine was produced primarily from the precursors phenyl-2-propanone and methylamine (the P-2-P method).[5,8] The combination of a crack down by the Department of Justice on West Coast gangs and the Controlled Substances Act of 1970, which made the ingredients of the P-2-P method controlled substances, resulted in a shift in the manufacturing and distribution of methamphetamine to small makeshift laboratories.

In the 1980s, a crystalline form of methamphetamine that could be smoked, called ice, began to be imported from Asia to Hawaii.[10] This highly addictive form of methamphetamine quickly found its way to the US West Coast and slowly began working it way east[11]; by 1990, methamphetamine had replaced cocaine as the stimulant of choice among drug users in many areas of California.[12] What would ultimately propel methamphetamine abuse to the forefront of the DEA war on drugs, and to the front pages of mainstream magazines and newspapers, was the rural meth lab. Unlike the cultivation of the coca leaf or opium poppy, the manufacture of methamphetamine is not limited by geographic location. By using OTC ephedrine and pseudoephedrine as the main precursors, making methamphetamine became simpler and more efficient. Methamphetamine laboratories manufacturing relatively pure crystal methamphetamine began to pop up across the Midwest; with the small investment of approximately $200, a methamphetamine cook could easily earn between $2000 and $5000.[13] Despite the relative simplicity of its synthesis (by traditional chemistry standards), cooking methamphetamine requires heating volatile hydrocarbons. When done by those without chemistry backgrounds and, as it often is, in poorly ventilated areas, fires and explosions can ensue. In fact, many methamphetamine laboratories have been discovered only after they have caught fire or exploded.[14,15] In an attempt to decrease the growing methamphetamine crisis, Congress passed the 2005 Combat Methamphetamine Epidemic Act, which limited access to pseudoephedrine. This limitation shut down vast numbers of small and medium-sized laboratories, resulting in a decline in the number of admissions for methamphetamine abuse in 2006—the first time in 10 years.[10]

With increasing numbers of large-scale manufacturers in Mexico, and other parts of the world, methamphetamine continues to be a significant problem in the United States. Because it has its most devastating effects on the central nervous system (CNS), it is important for neurologists to recognize signs of abuse and the many neurologic problems caused by methamphetamine. This article should help the practicing neurologist recognize and treat these patients, improving their chance to function drug free in society.

PHARMACOLOGY AND TOXICOLOGY

Both the acute and chronic neurologic effects of methamphetamine are the result of its pharmacology and toxicology. The acute effects of methamphetamine are those of the flight-or-fight response: increased heart rate and blood pressure, vasoconstriction, bronchodilation, and hyperglycemia.[16] In addition, methamphetamine causes CNS stimulation, which may result in euphoria, increased energy and alertness, intense curiosity and emotions, decreased anxiety, and enhanced self-esteem.[16]

Whether snorted, smoked, or injected, methamphetamine rapidly crosses the blood brain barrier where it can exert powerful effects on several neurochemical systems. Because of its lipophilic nature, methamphetamine has increased CNS penetration and is more potent than its parent compound, amphetamine.[17] Once in the CNS, it binds to dopamine, norepinephrine, and, to a lesser extent, serotonin transporters located on neuronal cell membranes; at higher concentrations, methamphetamine may also cross the cell membranes independent of transporter binding. Once bound, transporters pump methamphetamine into the neuron where it is taken up by vesicular monoamine transporters. The high pKa (pKa =10.1) of methamphetamine[18] disrupts the proton gradient, which normally keeps monoamines within the vesicle. This causes monamines to leave the vesicle and accumulate in the cytoplasm where they are reverse transported out of the cell through the same transporters that pumped methamphetamine into the cell.[19,20]

In addition to increasing their release, methamphetamine also decreases monoamine reuptake and enzyme degradation.[21] The net result is that methamphetamine causes a rapid and sustained increase in the extracellular concentrations of monoamines. One of the reasons methamphetamine has exceeded cocaine in worldwide usage is that it has a longer half-life (12 hours compared with 90 minutes) and, therefore, a much longer duration of action,[22] allowing the drug addict to have a longer and more sustained high. Although many receptors have been implicated in mediating the complex physiologic responses to amphetamines, the underlying clinical effects associated with methamphetamine use involve excessive stimulation of the sympathetic nervous system. It is the rapid and sustained activation of this system that is responsible for methamphetamine's recognizable adrenergic toxidrome: tachycardia, hypertension, mydriasis, diaphoresis, and psychomotor agitation. In addition, it is the prolonged release of central monoamines and activation of the sympathetic nervous system that is responsible for most of the acute neurologic complications associated with methamphetamine use (eg, strokes, seizures, agitation, and hyperthermia).[20,23,24] The sustained and repeated release of central monoamines is also largely to blame for the chronic neurologic effects of methamphetamine abuse.[20]

With repeated use in both humans and experimental animal models, methamphetamine depletes the brain's stores of dopamine and damages dopamine and serotonin nerve terminals. This may be a contributing factor to methamphetamine's high abuse potential; without the drug, users may have an impaired ability to experience pleasure (anhedonia), slipping into a deep depression. Based on current evidence, the complex mechanisms by which methamphetamine damages neurons involves increases in intracellular and extracellular concentrations of dopamine, which sets off a cascade of events, including oxidative stress, neuroinflammation, and excitatory neurotoxicity.[25]

It has also been shown that hyperthermia, a known complication of methamphetamine use, exacerbates this neurotoxicity.[25] Although this article focuses predominantly on methamphetamine, the similarities in the pharmacology, toxicology, and clinical effects between methamphetamine, amphetamine, and other stimulants (eg, cocaine and 3,4-methylenedioxmethamphemine [ecstasy]) makes the following discussions on neurologic complications largely translatable to other CNS stimulants.

NEUROPSYCHIATRIC COMPLICATIONS

Dopamine and serotonin neurons project widely throughout the CNS and are known to influence a variety of behaviors and functions. It should not be surprising that chronic methamphetamine abuse, which can damage dopamine and serotonin nerve terminals, is associated with deficits in neuropsychological testing. It has been estimated that 40% of methamphetamine users have abnormalities on neuropsychiatric tests.[26] In a well-done meta-analysis of studies examining the effects of chronic methamphetamine abuse on neuropsychiatric function, the most frequently reported deficits involve episodic memory, executive function, and motor function.[27] Of these, the greatest impairments are in episodic memory; this form of memory is thought to be the most susceptible to neuronal dysfunction.[28] As episodic memory allows one to consciously re-experience past events,[28] methamphetamine users who, by virtue of damaged episodic memory, forget past mistakes associated with their drug usage may be doomed to repeat them.

Another effect of chronic methamphetamine abuse is damage to executive function. With impaired executive function, methamphetamine abusers are likely to be distractible, impulsive, act inappropriately despite social cues to the contrary, and lack goals. In studies, patients addicted to methamphetamine prefer smaller, immediate rewards over larger, delayed rewards.[29] To overcome that wish for immediate rewards, addicts must activate the higher cognitive control systems, which, by virtue of their damaged executive system, is not an easy task for methamphetamine-dependent individuals.[29] Another consequence of impaired executive function, demonstrated in patients with damaged frontal lobes, is perseveration: the inability to change behavior even when the current behavior becomes destructive.[30] It is easy to imagine how damage to episodic memory and executive function might result in continued methamphetamine abuse despite the physical and emotional toil it reaps on users and their families. By chemically converting users into a modern Phineas Gage, methamphetamine exerts a powerful influence on behavior and decision making. Although not specifically tested, it is also possible that persons with damaged episodic memory and executive function, before using drugs, may be more susceptible to drug abuse and addiction and may have a greater risk for relapse.

Although studies show motor deficits in chronic methamphetamine abusers, these deficits do not typically involve gross movements, as with Parkinson's disease, but rather affect fine-motor dexterity (eg, placing pegs in a pegboard). These deficits would seem to be in line with studies showing that damage to dopamine terminals is more prevalent in the caudate (more involved in cognitive motor activities) then the putamen (more involved in pure motor activities) regions of the basal ganglia.[31,32]

Along with neuropsychiatric deficits, methamphetamine abusers suffer from mental illnesses, with anxiety,[33–35] depression,[27,35–37] and psychosis[22,27,37,38] being the most commonly reported. Of these, the neurologist is perhaps most likely to be confronted with patients suffering from psychosis.

After World War II, Japan suffered not only from a methamphetamine epidemic but also from an epidemic of drug-induced psychosis.[39–42] It has been estimated that at its height (between 1945–1955), there were as many as 200,000 persons in Japan with drug-induced psychosis.[42] Although much of the research on methamphetamine-induced psychosis has been conducted in Japan, similar reports have been reported in the United States and other countries.[43,44]

The symptoms of methamphetamine-induced psychosis are similar to those seen with schizophrenia; the most frequently reported symptoms are delusions of persecution and auditory hallucinations.[39–42,44–46] Although not as commonly reported, negative symptoms (eg, poverty of speech and psychomotor retardation) have also been seen with methamphetamine-induced psychosis.[44] In addition to a similar symptomatology, both schizophrenia and amphetamine-evoked psychosis can be effectively treated with dopamine antagonists.[47] The similarities between these disorders have lead many researchers to use amphetamines to model schizophrenia in laboratory animals.[42,48]

The development of psychosis is more readily seen in people using higher methamphetamine concentrations for prolonged periods of time.[39,45,46,49,50] The reported doses required, duration of abuse, and onset of symptoms are highly variable, as is the duration of psychotic symptoms (from 1 week to an indefinite duration).[16,51] Even if symptoms abate with abstinence, they can reemerge with repeat usage or under stressful situations.[40] One of the debates associated with psychosis and methamphetamine is whether it is the result of methamphetamine-induced neurotoxicity (ie, altered dopaminergic neurotransmission) or whether the 2 disorders coexist so that persons with mental illness are more likely to abuse methamphetamine (so-called dual diagnosis). The later seems to be supported by data showing that persons with predispositions to mental illness, such as strong family histories, are significantly more likely to develop methamphetamine-associated psychosis.[49,50] Furthermore, schizophrenics given low doses of methamphetamine will have exacerbations of their symptoms.[52] Therefore, it has been suggested that in susceptible individuals methamphetamine abuse may be a trigger that unmasks schizophrenia/psychosis.[53] Others have suggested that persons with schizophrenia/psychosis seek out illicit drugs as a form of self-treatment,[54] or, as recent data suggests, that neuronal deficits underlying the development of schizophrenia make individuals more prone to develop drug addiction.[55] Either way, it is clear that methamphetamine abuse can result in the development of acute and, in some cases, chronic psychosis and that practicing neurologists should be aware of this association. With the significant increase in the number of persons abusing methamphetamine, it remains to be seen if there will be a concomitant rise in patients requiring treatment for psychosis.

FORMICATION

One interesting aspect of chronic methamphetamine psychosis is the delusion of parasitosis or formication (the thought that one is infested with and being bitten by bugs).[43,46,56–59] Commonly known as *meth mites*, this is a frequent complaint in heavy daily users of methamphetamine. In studies of patients admitted to drug treatment facilities for methamphetamine abuse, approximately 40% of the patients report having had formication[43,46]; if the patients had ever suffered from psychosis, then the percentage of persons experiencing formication rose to 70%.[46] It is interesting that similar symptoms have been reported in animals chronically administered d-amphetamine.[57,58,60] These delusions may cause patients to repetitively pick at their skin resulting in scarring of their face and extremities.[59,61] Constant picking combined with neglect of hygiene also increase the risk for developing skin infections, including abscesses and cellulitis from methicillin-resistant *Staphylococcus aureus*.[62] Along with abstinence from drug usage, dopamine antagonists have been shown to help patients with drug-induced formication.[57] Although formication is not unique to methamphetamine (it has also been reported with cocaine[63] and schizophrenia[57]), the finding of multiple pockmarks on a patient's face and extremities, or recurrent skin abscesses in these areas, should increase a clinician's suspicion of chronic methamphetamine abuse.

STEREOTYPY OR PUNDING

One of the unique manifestations of methamphetamine abuse is the development of punding. The word *punding* is Swedish for "blockhead."[64,65] It was first coined by Rylander, who learned of the slang term from chronic amphetamine and phenmetrazine (another stimulant abused in Sweden in the 1960s) users as they described the abnormal persistent behaviors displayed by themselves and other addicts.[64] Punding has since become a term for non–goal-directed repetitive activity. Patient-reported examples include assembling and disassembling clocks and watches or incessantly sorting through purses. What makes these behaviors troublesome is the duration of time users would dedicate to such tasks without any apparent gain. There seems to be a predilection for punding to entail activities that users had previously been involved with. For example, a carpenter abusing amphetamines may repetitively build wooden objects; artists may doodle, paint, or draw excessively; a businessman may make and add to spreadsheets for hours.[66] There is also a gender-related component: men typically tinkering with electronics and women more commonly involved in grooming behaviors, such as hair brushing and nail polishing.[64,65,67–69] It is interesting that stereotyped repetitive movements, such as head bobbing, licking, gnawing, and sniffing, are also seen in a variety of animals given amphetamines.[70]

Although first reported in amphetamine abusers, punding has also been reported in cocaine users[71] and, more recently, in patients with Parkinson's disease receiving dopamine replacement therapy.[66,67] Similar to chronic stimulant abusers, patients with Parkinson's disease have dysfunctional dopaminergic neurotransmission and can develop psychosis.[67] This finding suggests a similar pathophysiologic mechanism. Although few controlled studies have been done on punding with substance abuse, there is some data available on its incidence. In a study of 50 patients addicted to cocaine, Fasano reported that 38% had some form of punding.[66] These patients spent, on average, 3 hours a day engaged in their repetitive activities.[66] One patient reported spending up to 14 hours a day playing computer games and collecting things.[67] It is interesting that the majority of interviewed patients in this study reported that their behavior began shortly after their first drug usage. In addition, the duration and amount of drug use did not seem to predict which users would develop punding and which would not.[67] This finding suggests that, like the development of stimulant-induced psychosis, there may be a predisposition for the development of punding that is merely brought out by the drug. As previously discussed, the same abnormal brain circuitry that increases one's risk for becoming addicted may also be involved in the development of such stereotyped behaviors. In his first report on the topic, Rylander described punding in 26% (40 of 150) of the amphetamine addicts he interviewed.[64] These patients shared identical symptomatology as the cocaine addicts and patients with Parkinson's disease who engaged in punding. The majority of the drug addicts did not describe associated anxiety or distress over their activities, but thought of them with amusement. Some even found them pleasurable. When abstaining from drug usage, punding typically abates. Although the neurologic mechanisms behind punding are not yet well delineated, it appears to involve dopamine. Repeated dosing of amphetamines in animals results in behavioral sensitization. This sensitization is manifested as increased locomotion and stereotypic behavior with each subsequent dose of amphetamine. This sensitization appears to involve both glutamate and dopamine, and, more recently, dopamine-mediated decreases in acetylcholine have been implicated.[67,72,73] As concentrations of extracellular dopamine increase with each subsequent dose of amphetamine, one could envision over time this excess dopamine causing neurotoxicity or change the normal balance between dopamine 1 (D1) and dopamine 2 (D2) receptor activity[52]; In a review on the topic, Fasano makes a strong argument for the involvement of both D1 and D2 receptors in the development of punding, and suggests that, if needed, treatments might include atypical antipsychotics.[66]

CHRONIC METHAMPHETAMINE ABUSE AND THE DEVELOPMENT OF PARKINSON'S DISEASE

People with Parkinson's disease[66,67] also exhibit unusual impulse-control disorders and punding. Similar to methamphetamine abusers, patients with Parkinson's disease, whether they are newly diagnosed[74] or have had dopamine-replacement therapies,[75] have gender-specific compulsivity problems. Men more frequently suffer from pathologic gambling and compulsive sexual behavior, whereas women tend toward compulsive buying and binge eating. The collective animal and human data clearly show that high-dose methamphetamine abuse causes alterations in striatal dopaminergic neurotransmission. Numerous pathology and imaging studies have shown reductions in striatal dopamine, tyrosine hydroxylase, and dopamine transporters.[6,32,76–80] Because these findings are also found in persons with Parkinson's disease, it is logical to expect that chronic methamphetamine addicts would develop signs of Parkinson's disease.

The current and prevailing theory is that abusing methamphetamine does not increase one's risk of developing Parkinson's disease or Parkinsonism.[31,32,76] Several hypotheses have been put forth to explain the discrepancy between the research and clinical data.[31,32,76] The simplest hypothesis is that they are different disorders. Parkinson's disease involves loss of dopaminergic neurons in the substantia nigra, whereas methamphetamine abuse causes alterations in dopaminergic nerve terminals, but not in the cell bodies themselves.[32] In studies of methamphetamine abusers, the reductions in dopamine have a different distribution than in patients with Parkinson's disease. Methamphetamine users have greater dopamine reductions in the caudate compared with the putamen, with patients with Parkinson's disease showing the opposite.[32] Another hypothesis is that once users become drug abstinent, the damaged dopaminergic nerve terminals begin to recover; decreases in dopamine transporters of methamphetamine abusers were found to significantly recover with prolonged (>12 months) abstinence.[79]

Another hypothesis is that methamphetamine abusers do not actually damage their dopaminergic nerve terminals, and that the findings of reduce dopamine levels represent a compensatory response to repeated elevations in monoamines. The strongest argument for this has been that the vesicular transporter-2 (VMAT2), which is known to be reduced in Parkinson's disease and to be resistant to drug-compensatory regulation, is not significantly reduced in abstinent methamphetamine abusers.[6,81] In fact, a more recent positron emission tomography (PET) study of nonabstinent methamphetamine abusers found increases in VMAT2.[82] This finding was thought to be caused by reductions in vesicular dopamine, depleted from recent release, resulting in less dopamine being available to compete for binding to VMAT2.[82]

Another intriguing hypothesis involves nicotine and nicotine receptors. Acetylcholine nicotinic mechanisms can influence the behavioral and neurochemical effects of psychomotor stimulant drugs and vice versa.[83] An overwhelming number of methamphetamine users smoke cigarettes compared with the general population (87%–92% vs 22%).[84] Because cigarette smoking negatively correlates with development of Parkinson's disease,[85] methamphetamine abusers may be protected or self-treated.[31]

Some researchers think that methamphetamine abuse does increase the risk for developing Parkinson's disease.[76,86,87] One retrospective study, looking at hospital admissions over a 10-year period, found an increased incidence of Parkinson's disease among patients who had a prior history of being admitted with a methamphetamine-related problem.[87] Because it may take many years before reductions in dopamine reach the levels mediating clinical symptoms, it is possible that the patients enrolled in many of the prospective clinical studies are not old enough to show symptoms; the majority of studies involve young adults. What instead may occur is that as methamphetamine use increases in young adults, we may see a shift in the age of onset of Parkinson's disease. There have been 2 studies involving the same group of patients that support this idea. In a phone survey of patients with Parkinson's disease receiving care at 1 of 3 clinics, patients with Parkinson's disease were significantly more likely (odds ratio = 8, confidence interval 1.6–41.4) to have used amphetamines than their unaffected spouses,[88] and in the majority of these patients, their exposures to amphetamines occurred years (~27) before symptoms onset.[88] Compared with patients with Parkinson's disease without a history of exposure, those patients with a history of amphetamine use were significantly younger at the age of symptom onset, but not at the age of diagnosis.[86] This study is small, however, and subject, by its design, to recall bias. Further work is needed to confirm whether there is, in fact, an association between amphetamine use and the development of Parkinson's disease.

CHOREOATHETOID MOVEMENTS AND DYSKINESIAS

A potential complication of methamphetamine-induced damage to the dopaminergic nervous system is the development of dyskinesias and choreoathetoid movements.[89] There have been numerous reports of choreoathetoid movements (involuntary purposeless and uncontrollable movements with features of both chorea and athetosis) in patients using or abusing amphetamines.[46,68,69,90–94] In one report, patients with underlying chorea (Sydenham, Huntington, and Lupus) were given an intravenous dose of amphetamine to assess its effect on their baseline movements. In each of these patients, amphetamine dramatically worsened their underlying chorea.[95] The increases in limb movements provoked by amphetamines could be prevented if patients were pretreated with the D2 antagonist haloperidol.[95] Because a group of control patients without chorea that were given amphetamine did not develop movement disorders, the investigators suggested that the development of chorea from amphetamines may require a underlying damage to the striatum.[95] This supposition would seem to be supported from several lines of evidence. For one, numerous studies have shown that methamphetamine abusers have evidence of dopaminergic neurotoxicity in the striatum.[6,25,96] Additionally, chronic methamphetamine abusers, even without frank chorea, often have demonstrable movement disorders.[97] Furthermore, in some patients, movement disorders can last for years even after they have stopped using amphetamines.[64,68] Lastly, patients who have stopped abusing amphetamine, and subsequently recovered from their choreoathetoid movement disorder, will often redevelop symptoms the first time they use amphetamines again, suggesting that patients may become permanently susceptible.[68]

The description of choreoathetoid movements typically involves the limbs, neck, and face and often has a rhythmic dancelike quality. Similar to other dyskinesias, symptoms disappear while patients sleep.[68] Although in some patients dopamine antagonists and benzodiazepines have been found to relieve symptoms,[69,91,95] in others they have had no benefit.[68] Not limited to amphetamines, choreoathetoid movements have also been reported with other stimulants, including cocaine (known as crack dancing).[64,97–99] Although the paucity of literature on this topic suggests that the development of these symptoms is rare, the fact that there are street names for this in English and Spanish suggests that it may occur more commonly than reported.[98] It is a sad and real possibility that, among other reasons, many of the homeless persons seen dancing and writhing around on the street corners of many major cities may be manifesting signs of stimulant-induced choreoathetoid movements.

DENTAL CARIES

Although not traditionally considered a neurologic complication, the development of dental caries and teeth erosion in chronic methamphetamine abusers may be the result of elevations in brain monoamines. Referred to as *meth mouth*, advanced dental caries, tooth loss, and tooth fractures seen among methamphetamine users is the result of decreased saliva production (xerostomia) combined with teeth grinding (bruxism) and jaw clenching.[100–108] Additional contributors to methamphetamine-related tooth decay include poor oral hygiene combined with the consumption of sugar-containing carbonated soft drinks, which is a common habit among methamphetamine users, with Mountain Dew being their drink of choice.[100–102,106,109] Dental caries seen with meth mouth occur in a similar pattern to other disorders involving xerostomia (eg, Sjögren and radiation), involving the buccal smooth surface of the posterior teeth and the interproximal areas of the anterior teeth.[100,102] Decay can progress to complete destruction of dental enamel, with many young methamphetamine addicts requiring dentures.[110] The mechanism of methamphetamine-induced xerostomia appears to be mediated by central alpha-2 receptors, which, when bound by norepinephrine, decreases salivary flow.[103,109,111] Along with increasing dopamine, methamphetamine causes sustained increases in extracellular concentrations of norepinephrine.[112] Although the cause of bruxism is not well known, it is thought to be of central origin and, likewise, to involve central monoamines.[107,108,113] Unlike nocturnal bruxism, methamphetamine users will often have bruxism day and night.[107,108] Although the practicing neurologist is unlikely to be consulted to see patients because of dental caries, recognizing the dental and dermatologic manifestations of chronic methamphetamine abuse may help to identify at-risk patients.

SUMMARY

Chronic methamphetamine abuse has devastating effects on the CNS. The degree to which addicts will tolerate the dysfunction in the way they think, feel, move, and even look, is a powerful testimony to the addictive properties of this drug. Although the mechanisms behind these disorders are complex, at their heart they involve the recurring increase in the concentrations of central monoamines with subsequent dysfunction in dopaminergic neurotransmission. The mainstay of treatment for the problems associated with chronic methamphetamine abuse is abstinence. However, by recognizing the manifestations of chronic abuse, clinicians will be better able to help their patients get treatment for their addiction and to deal with the neurologic complications related to chronic abuse.

ACKNOWLEDGMENTS

The author would like to acknowledge the valuable editorial assistance of Pamela J. Durant.

REFERENCES

1. Streatfeild D. Cocaine: an unauthorized biography. New York: Picador; 2001.
2. Nagai T, Kamiyama S. Forensic toxicologic analysis of methamphetamine and amphetamine optical isomers by high performance liquid chromatography. Int J Legal Med 1988;101:151–9.
3. Nagai H. Studies on the components of *Ephedraceae* in herb medicine. Yahugaku Zasshi 1893;139:901–33.
4. Miller MA. History and epidemiology of amphetamine abuse in the United States. In: Klee H, editor. Amphetamine misuse: international perspectives on current trends. Reading (UK): Harwood Academic Publishers; 1997. p. 113–33.
5. Anglin MD, Burke C, Perrochet B, et al. History of the methamphetamine problem. J Psychoactive Drugs 2000;32:137–41.
6. Wilson JM, Kalasinsky KS, Levey AI, et al. Striatal dopamine nerve terminal markers in human, chronic methamphetamine users. Nat Med 1996;2:699–703.

7. Suwaki H, Fukui S, Konuma K. Methamphetamine abuse in Japan: its 45 year history and the current situation. In: Klee H, editor. Amphetamine misuse: international perspectives on current trends. Reading (UK): Harwood Academic Publishers; 1997.

8. Hunt D, Kuck S, Truitt L. Methamphetamine use: lessons learned: report to the National Institute of Justice. Cambridge (MA): Abt Associates Inc; 2006. Available at: http://www.ncjrs.gov/pdffiles1/nij/grants/209730.pdf. Accessed May 10, 2011.

9. UNDOC. Annual Report 2008. 2008. Available at: www.unodc.org/documents/about-unodc/AR08_WEB.pdf. Accessed January 19, 2011.

10. Gonzales R, Mooney L, Rawson RA. The Methamphetamine Problem in the United States. Annu Rev Public Health 2010;31:385–98.

11. Office of National Drug Control Policy. II. America's Drug Use Profile. Available at: http://www.ncjrs.gov/ondcppubs/publications/policy/ndcs01/chap2.html. Accessed January 19, 2011.

12. Derlet RW, Heischober B. Methamphetamine. Stimulant of the 1990s? West J Med 1990;153:625–8.

13. Costs of Meth. Available at: http://www5.semo.edu/criminal/medfels/text_meth_cost.htm. Accessed January 19, 2011.

14. Denehy J. The meth epidemic: its effect on children and communities. J Sch Nurs 2006;22:63–5.

15. Betsinger G. Coping with meth lab hazards. Occup Health Saf 2006;75:50, 52, 54–8, passim.

16. Cruickshank CC, Dyer KR. A review of the clinical pharmacology of methamphetamine. Addiction 2009;104:1085–99.

17. Lake CR, Quirk RS. CNS stimulants and look-alike drugs. Psychiatr Clin North Am 1984;7:689–701.

18. Brandle E, Fritzsch G, Greven J. Affinity of different local anesthetic drugs and catecholamines for the contraluminal transport system for organic cations in proximal tubules of rat kidneys. J Pharmacol Exp Ther 1992;260:734–41.

19. Fleckenstein AE, Volz TJ, Riddle EL, et al. New insights into the mechanism of action of amphetamines. Annu Rev Pharmacol Toxicol 2007;47:681–98.

20. Schep LJ, Slaughter RJ, Beasley DM. The clinical toxicology of metamfetamine. Clin Toxicol (Phila) 2010;48:675–94.

21. Suzuki O, Hattori H, Asano M, et al. Inhibition of monoamine oxidase by d-methamphetamine. Biochem Pharmacol 1980;29:2071–3.

22. Meredith CW, Jaffe C, Ang-Lee K, et al. Implications of chronic methamphetamine use: a literature review. Harv Rev Psychiatry 2005;13:141–54.

23. O'Connor AD, Rusyniak DE, Bruno A. Cerebrovascular and cardiovascular complications of alcohol and sympathomimetic drug abuse. Med Clin North Am 2005;89:1343–58.

24. Rusyniak DE, Sprague JE. Hyperthermic syndromes induced by toxins. Clin Lab Med 2006;26:165–84.

25. Yamamoto BK, Moszczynska A, Gudelsky GA. Amphetamine toxicities. Ann N Y Acad Sci 2010;1187:101–21.

26. Rippeth JD, Heaton RK, Carey CL, et al. Methamphetamine dependence increases risk of neuropsychological impairment in HIV infected persons. J Int Neuropsychol Soc 2004;10:1–14.

27. Scott JC, Woods SP, Matt GE, et al. Neurocognitive effects of methamphetamine: a critical review and meta-analysis. Neuropsychol Rev 2007;17:275–97.

28. Tulving E. Episodic memory: from mind to brain. Annu Rev Psychol 2002;53:1–25.

29. Hoffman WF, Schwartz DL, Huckans MS, et al. Cortical activation during delay discounting in abstinent methamphetamine dependent individuals. Psychopharmacology (Berl) 2008;201:183–93.

30. Gilbert SJ, Burgess PW. Executive function. Curr Biol 2008;18:R110–4.

31. Caligiuri MP, Buitenhuys C. Do preclinical findings of methamphetamine-induced motor abnormalities translate to an observable clinical phenotype? Neuropsychopharmacology 2005;30:2125–34.

32. Moszczynska A, Fitzmaurice P, Ang L, et al. Why is parkinsonism not a feature of human methamphetamine users? Brain 2004;127(Pt 2):363–70.

33. Glasner-Edwards S, Mooney LJ, Marinelli-Casey P, et al. Anxiety disorders among methamphetamine dependent adults: association with post-treatment functioning. Am J Addict 2010;19:385–90.

34. Hall W, Hando J, Darke S, et al. Psychological morbidity and route of administration among amphetamine users in Sydney, Australia. Addiction 1996;91:81–7.

35. McKetin R, Ross J, Kelly E, et al. Characteristics and harms associated with injecting versus smoking methamphetamine among methamphetamine treatment entrants. Drug Alcohol Rev 2008;27:277–85.

36. Copeland AL, Sorensen JL. Differences between methamphetamine users and cocaine users in treatment. Drug Alcohol Depend 2001;62:91–5.

37. Newton TF, Kalechstein AD, Duran S, et al. Methamphetamine abstinence syndrome: preliminary findings. Am J Addict 2004;13:248–55.

38. Nordahl TE, Salo R, Leamon M. Neuropsychological effects of chronic methamphetamine use on neurotransmitters and cognition: a review. J Neuropsychiatry Clin Neurosci 2003;15:317–35.

39. Iwanami A, Sugiyama A, Kuroki N, et al. Patients with methamphetamine psychosis admitted to a psychiatric hospital in Japan. A preliminary report. Acta Psychiatr Scand 1994;89:428–32.

40. Sato M. A lasting vulnerability to psychosis in patients with previous methamphetamine psychosis. Ann N Y Acad Sci 1992;654:160–70.

41. Shimazono Y, Matsushima E. Behavioral and neuroimaging studies on schizophrenia in Japan. Psychiatry Clin Neurosci 1995;49:3–11.

42. Yui K, Ikemoto S, Ishiguro T, et al. Studies of amphetamine or methamphetamine psychosis in Japan: relation of methamphetamine psychosis to schizophrenia. Ann N Y Acad Sci 2000;914:1–12.

43. Hawks D, Mitcheson M, Ogborne A, et al. Abuse of methylamphetamine. Br Med J 1969;2:715–21.

44. Srisurapanont M, Ali R, Marsden J, et al. Psychotic symptoms in methamphetamine psychotic in-patients. Int J Neuropsychopharmacol 2003;6:347–52.

45. Mahoney JJ 3rd, Kalechstein AD, De La Garza R 2nd, et al. Presence and persistence of psychotic symptoms in cocaine- versus methamphetamine-dependent participants. Am J Addict 2008;17:83–98.

46. Ellinwood EH. Amphetamine Psychosis: I. Description of the individuals and process. J Nerv Ment Dis 1967;144:273–83.

47. Angrist B, Lee HK, Gershon S. The antagonism of amphetamine-induced symptomatology by a neuroleptic. Am J Psychiatry 1974;131:817–9.

48. Snyder SH. Amphetamine psychosis: a "model" schizophrenia mediated by catecholamines. Am J Psychiatry 1973;130:61–7.

49. Chen CK, Lin SK, Sham PC, et al. Pre-morbid characteristics and co-morbidity of methamphetamine users with and without psychosis. Psychol Med 2003;33:1407–14.

50. Chen CK, Lin SK, Sham PC, et al. Morbid risk for psychiatric disorder among the relatives of methamphetamine users with and without psychosis. Am J Med Genet 2005;136B:87–91.

51. Bell DS. The experimental reproduction of amphetamine psychosis. Arch Gen Psychiatry 1973;29:35–40.

52. Lieberman JA, Kinon BJ, Loebel AD. Dopaminergic mechanisms in idiopathic and drug-induced psychoses. Schizophr Bull 1990;16:97–110.

53. Bell DS. Comparison of amphetamine psychosis and schizophrenia. Br J Psychiatry 1965;111:701–7.

54. Buckley PF. Substance abuse in schizophrenia: a review. J Clin Psychiatry 1998; 59(Suppl 3):26–30.

55. Chambers RA, Krystal JH, Self DW. A neurobiological basis for substance abuse comorbidity in schizophrenia. Biol Psychiatry 2001;50:71–83.

56. Richards JR, Bretz SW, Johnson EB, et al. Methamphetamine abuse and emergency department utilization. West J Med 1999;170:198–202.

57. de Leon J, Antelo RE, Simpson G. Delusion of parasitosis or chronic tactile hallucinosis: hypothesis about their brain physiopathology. Compr Psychiatry 1992; 33:25–33.

58. Ellinwood EH, Sudilovsky A. Chronic amphetamine intoxication: behavioral model of psychoses. In: Cole JO, Freedman AM, Friedhoff AJ, editors. Psychopathology and psychopharmacology. Baltimore (MD): Johns Hopkins University Press; 1972. p. 51–70.

59. Yaffee HS. Cutaneous stigmas associated with Methedrine (methamphetamine). Arch Dermatol 1971;104:687.

60. Ellison GD, Eison MS. Continuous amphetamine intoxication: an animal model of the acute psychotic episode. Psychol Med 1983;13:751–61.

61. Liu SW, Lien MH, Fenske NA. The effects of alcohol and drug abuse on the skin. Clin Dermatol 2010;28:391–9.

62. Cohen AL, Shuler C, McAllister S, et al. Methamphetamine use and methicillin-resistant *Staphylococcus aureus* skin infections. Emerg Infect Dis 2007;13: 1707–13.

63. Siegel RK. Cocaine hallucinations. Am J Psychiatry 1978;135:309–14.

64. Rylander G. Psychoses and the punding and choreiform syndromes in addiction to central stimulant drugs. Psychiatr Neurol Neurochir 1972;75:203–12.

65. Schiorring E. Psychopathology induced by "speed drugs". Pharmacol Biochem Behav 1981;14(Suppl 1):109–22.

66. Fasano A, Petrovic I. Insights into pathophysiology of punding reveal possible treatment strategies. Mol Psychiatry 2010;15:560–73.

67. O'Sullivan SS, Evans AH, Lees AJ. Dopamine dysregulation syndrome: an overview of its epidemiology, mechanisms and management. CNS Drugs 2009;23: 157–70.

68. Lundh H, Tunving K. An extrapyramidal choreiform syndrome caused by amphetamine addiction. J Neurol Neurosurg Psychiatry 1981;44:728–30.

69. Rhee KJ, Albertson TE, Douglas JC. Choreoathetoid disorder associated with amphetamine-like drugs. Am J Emerg Med 1988;6:131–3.

70. Randrup A, Munkvad I. Stereotyped activities produced by amphetamine in several animal species and man. Psychopharmacologia 1967;11:300–10.

71. Fasano A, Barra A, Nicosia P, et al. Cocaine addiction: from habits to stereotypical-repetitive behaviors and punding. Drug Alcohol Depend 2008;96:178–82.

72. Aliane V, Perez S, Bohren Y, et al. Key role of striatal cholinergic interneurons in processes leading to arrest of motor stereotypies. Brain 2010;134:110–8.

73. Pierce RC, Kalivas PW. A circuitry model of the expression of behavioral sensitization to amphetamine-like psychostimulants. Brain Res Brain Res Rev 1997; 25:192–216.

74. Antonini A, Siri C, Santangelo G, et al. Impulsivity and compulsivity in drug-naive patients with Parkinson's disease. Mov Disord 2011;26:464–8.

75. Weintraub D, Koester J, Potenza MN, et al. Impulse control disorders in Parkinson disease: a cross-sectional study of 3090 patients. Arch Neurol 2010;67:589–95.

76. Guilarte TR. Is methamphetamine abuse a risk factor in parkinsonism? Neurotoxicology 2001;22:725–31.

77. McCann UD, Kuwabara H, Kumar A, et al. Persistent cognitive and dopamine transporter deficits in abstinent methamphetamine users. Synapse 2008;62: 91–100.

78. Truong JG. Age-dependent methamphetamine-induced alterations in vesicular monoamine transporter-2 function: implications for neurotoxicity. J Pharmacol Exp Ther 2005;314:1087–92.

79. Volkow ND, Chang L, Wang GJ, et al. Loss of dopamine transporters in methamphetamine abusers recovers with protracted abstinence. J Neurosci 2001;21: 9414–8.

80. Volkow ND, Chang L, Wang GJ, et al. Association of dopamine transporter reduction with psychomotor impairment in methamphetamine abusers. Am J Psychiatry 2001;158:377–82.

81. Johanson CE, Frey KA, Lundahl LH, et al. Cognitive function and nigrostriatal markers in abstinent methamphetamine abusers. Psychopharmacology (Berl) 2006;185:327–38.

82. Boileau I, Rusjan P, Houle S, et al. Increased vesicular monoamine transporter binding during early abstinence in human methamphetamine users: is VMAT2 a stable dopamine neuron biomarker? J Neurosci 2008;28:9850–6.

83. Desai RI, Bergman J. Drug discrimination in methamphetamine-trained rats: effects of cholinergic nicotinic compounds. J Pharmacol Exp Ther 2010;335: 807–16.

84. Weinberger AH, Sofuoglu M. The impact of cigarette smoking on stimulant addiction. Am J Drug Alcohol Abuse 2009;35:12–7.

85. Hernán MA, Takkouche B, Caamaño-Isorna F, et al. A meta-analysis of coffee drinking, cigarette smoking, and the risk of Parkinson's disease. Ann Neurol 2002;52:276–84.

86. Christine CW, Garwood ER, Schrock LE, et al. Parkinsonism in patients with a history of amphetamine exposure. Mov Disord 2010;25:228–31.

87. Callaghan RC, Cunningham JK, Sajeev G, et al. Incidence of Parkinson's disease among hospital patients with methamphetamine-use disorders. Mov Disord 2010; 25:2333–9.

88. Garwood ER, Bekele W, McCulloch CE, et al. Amphetamine exposure is elevated in Parkinson's disease. Neurotoxicology 2006;27:1003–6.

89. Janavs JL, Aminoff MJ. Dystonia and chorea in acquired systemic disorders. J Neurol Neurosurg Psychiatry 1998;65:436–45.

90. Shanson B. Amphetamine poisoning. Br Med J 1956;1(4966):576.

91. Downes MA, Whyte IM. Amphetamine-induced movement disorder. Emerg Med Australas 2005;17:277–80.

92. Mattson RH, Calverley JR. Dextroamphetamine-sulfate-induced dyskinesias. JAMA 1968;204:400–2.

93. Morgan JC, Winter WC, Wooten GF. Amphetamine-induced chorea in attention deficit-hyperactivity disorder. Mov Disord 2004;19:840–2.

94. Sperling LS, Horowitz JL. Methamphetamine-induced choreoathetosis and rhabdomyolysis. Ann Intern Med 1994;121:986.
95. Klawans HL, Weiner WJ. The effect of d-amphetamine on choreiform movement disorders. Neurology 1974;24:312–8.
96. Volkow ND, Chang L, Wang GJ, et al. Low level of brain dopamine D2 receptors in methamphetamine abusers: association with metabolism in the orbitofrontal cortex. Am J Psychiatry 2001;158:2015–21.
97. Bartzokis G, Beckson M, Wirshing DA, et al. Choreoathetoid movements in cocaine dependence. Biol Psychiatry 1999;45:1630–5.
98. Daras M, Koppel BS, Atos-Radzion E. Cocaine-induced choreoathetoid movements ('crack dancing'). Neurology 1994;44:751–2.
99. Stork CM, Cantor R. Pemoline induced acute choreoathetosis: case report and review of the literature. J Toxicol Clin Toxicol 1997;35:105–8.
100. Klasser GD, Epstein J. Methamphetamine and its impact on dental care. J Can Dent Assoc 2005;71:759–62.
101. ADA. Methamphetamine use and oral health. J Am Dent Assoc 2005;136:1491.
102. Shaner JW, Kimmes N, Saini T, et al. "Meth mouth": rampant caries in methamphetamine abusers. AIDS Patient Care STDS 2006;20:146–50.
103. Saini T, Edwards PC, Kimmes NS, et al. Etiology of xerostomia and dental caries among methamphetamine abusers. Oral Health Prev Dent 2005;3:189–95.
104. Donaldson M, Goodchild JH. Oral health of the methamphetamine abuser. Am J Health Syst Pharm 2006;63:2078–82.
105. Richards JR, Brofeldt BT. Patterns of tooth wear associated with methamphetamine use. J Periodontol 2000;71:1371–4.
106. Morio KA, Marshall TA, Qian F, et al. Comparing diet, oral hygiene and caries status of adult methamphetamine users and nonusers: a pilot study. J Am Dent Assoc 2008;139:171–6.
107. Winocur E, Gavish A, Voikovitch M, et al. Drugs and bruxism: a critical review. J Orofac Pain 2003;17:99–111.
108. Winocur E, Gavish A, Volfin G, et al. Oral motor parafunctions among heavy drug addicts and their effects on signs and symptoms of temporomandibular disorders. J Orofac Pain 2001;15:56–63.
109. Di Cugno F, Perec CJ, Tocci AA. Salivary secretion and dental caries experience in drug addicts. Arch Oral Biol 1981;26:363–7.
110. Shetty V, Mooney LJ, Zigler CM, et al. The relationship between methamphetamine use and increased dental disease. J Am Dent Assoc 2010;141:307–18.
111. Götrick B, Giglio D, Tobin G. Effects of amphetamine on salivary secretion. Eur J Oral Sci 2009;117:218–23.
112. Kuczenski R, Segal DS, Cho AK, et al. Hippocampus norepinephrine, caudate dopamine and serotonin, and behavioral responses to the stereoisomers of amphetamine and methamphetamine. J Neurosci 1995;15:1308–17.
113. Lobbezoo F, Naeije M. Bruxism is mainly regulated centrally, not peripherally. J Oral Rehabil 2001;28:1085–91.

Toxic Leukoencephalopathies

Laura M. Tormoehlen, MD[a,b,*]

KEYWORDS

- Post-anoxic • Carbon monoxide • Delayed neurologic sequelae • Heroin
- "Chasing the dragon" • Posterior reversible encephalopathy syndrome

COMMENTARY ON TOXIC LEUKOENCEPHALOPATHIES FOR PSYCHIATRIC PRACTICE

While these toxic leukoencephalopathies may present with acute, severe alteration of mental state necessitating hospital admission, they may also present with a more indolent subacute worsening of cognitive function resulting in primarily psychiatric symptoms. Thus, the psychiatrist may be the first evaluator of the patient. This is especially true of the delayed post-hypoxic leukoencephalopathy (DPHL), including the delayed neurologic sequelae (DNS) of carbon monoxide toxicity, because the mental state is normal or near-normal at hospital discharge, followed by onset of neuropsychiatric symptoms in the ensuing days to weeks. Many of these patients will have pre-existing psychiatric conditions, thus the manifestations of the leukoencephalopathy may mimic exacerbations of their known diagnoses. Similarly, the first stage of heroin inhalation leukoencephalopathy (HIL) is characterized by a primarily cerebellar syndrome with ataxia, pseudobulbar speech, apathy, and akathisia which may be attributed to underlying psychiatric disease and/or effects of psychiatric medications. Posterior reversible encephalopathy syndrome (PRES) may present initially to a psychiatrist in a patient with milder symptoms (headache, confusion, vision change), but PRES is more likely to present with an acute neurologic change, thus prompting emergency department evaluation.

This article originally appeared in the *August 2011 issue of Neurologic Clinics (Volume 29, Number 3)*.

The author has nothing to disclose.

[a] Department of Neurology, Indiana University School of Medicine, 545 Barnhill Drive, Indianapolis, IN 46202, USA; [b] Department of Emergency Medicine, Indiana University School of Medicine, 1701 North Senate Boulevard B401, Indianapolis, IN 46202, USA

* 1701 North Senate Boulevard, B417, Indianapolis, IN 46202.

E-mail address: laumjone@iupui.edu

http://dx.doi.org/10.1016/j.psc.2013.02.006
0193-953X/13/$ – see front matter © 2013 Elsevier Inc. All rights reserved.

psych.theclinics.com

KEY POINTS

- Diagnosis of each of these syndromes is made by thorough history and a high level of clinical suspicion, combined with neuroimaging.
- The imaging test of choice for each of these leukoencephalopathies is brain magnetic resonance imaging.
- Treatment for DPHL, including DNS, is symptomatic and supportive care. Hyperbaric oxygen for acute carbon monoxide poisoning, aimed at preventing DNS, remains controversial. Most patients will improve, but the degree of persistent cognitive deficit is variable.
- Treatment for HIL is largely supportive; however, there are reports of improvement with coenzyme Q, vitamin C and vitamin E.
- Treatment for PRES is removal of causative agents and measured blood pressure lowering.

Abbreviations for Toxic Leukoencephalopathies	
ADC	Apparent diffusion coefficient
CO poisoning	Carbon monoxide poisoning
DNS	Delayed neurologic sequelae
DPHL	Delayed posthypoxic leukoencephalopathy
DWI	Diffusion weighted imaging
FLAIR	Fluid-attenuated inversion recovery
HBOT	Hyperbaric oxygen therapy
PRES	Posterior reversible encephalopathy syndrome

Leukoencephalopathy is a syndrome of neurologic deficits, including alteration of mental status, caused by pathologic changes in the cerebral white matter. The term, *toxic leukoencephalopathy*, encompasses a wide variety of exposures and clinical presentations. The MRI findings in each of these entities is similar given the requisite involvement of the cerebral white matter but may be quite different in the distribution of areas involved, the extent of gray matter involvement, and findings on ancillary radiographic studies. The diagnosis in these syndromes is made by careful attention to the history, clinical features, and radiologic findings. The differential diagnosis of toxin-induced leukoencephalopathy includes multiple sclerosis, acute disseminated encephalomyelitis, progressive multifocal leukoencephalopathy, several rare leukodystrophies, gliomatosis cerebri, and encephalitis. The goal of this article is to give a detailed discussion of three of the best-defined toxic leukoencephalopathies: delayed posthypoxic leukoencephalopathy (DPHL), including delayed neurologic sequelae (DNS) of carbon monoxide (CO) poisoning; heroin inhalation leukoencephalopathy; and posterior reversible encephalopathy syndrome (PRES).

DELAYED POSTHYPOXIC LEUKOENCEPHALOPATHY

DPHL is a rare demyelinating syndrome that may occur after a prolonged period of poor cerebral oxygenation. The usual presentation is characterized by complete or near-complete recovery from the acute event, followed by onset of neuropsychologic symptoms days to weeks later. This pattern of symptomatology distinguishes it from acute hypoxic brain injury, which results in persistent effects and is associated with greater involvement of the gray matter.

Clinical Features

This phenomenon was first described in cases of CO toxicity[1] but has now been described in cases of cardiac arrest, complications of surgery and anesthesia, asphyxial gas poisoning, strangulation, shock, and respiratory depression from heroin or benzodiazepine overdose.[2–9]

Historically, DPHL is heralded by an acute event resulting in hypoxic insult. In all cases that are not associated with CO (discussed later), there is a period of unconsciousness or coma.[10] This is followed by neurologic recovery with subsequent return to usual activities. Then, after a period of days to weeks, there is acute deterioration with onset of neuropsychiatric symptoms that worsen over the course of a few days. Symptoms may include akinetic mutism (apathy, incontinence, mutism, and pseudobulbar affect) or parkinsonian features (tremor, gait and speech disturbance, rigidity, and masked facies), suggesting involvement of the white matter tracts of the frontal lobes and basal ganglia motor circuits, respectively.[2,11]

Radiologic Findings

Diffuse, confluent hypodensity of the white matter on CT of the head can be diagnostic if the clinical history suggests the possibility of DPHL. If the history is not clear or other diagnoses are possible, MRI is necessary to entertain the diagnosis. Classic MRI findings are T2-sequence hyperintense lesions in the periventricular white matter of the cerebral hemispheres with relative sparing of the cerebellum and brainstem. The lesions are typically nonenhancing and do not extend into the cortex. MR spectroscopy in DPHL patients has been reported to show an elevated choline peak, indicative of lipid membrane turnover and suggestive of demyelination.[12,13]

Pathophysiology and Pathologic Findings

The clinical event preceding DPHL produces a mild-to-moderate hypoxia. Severe hypoxia is more likely to result in acute, persistent hypoxic brain injury. Because the gray matter is more susceptible to acute severe hypoxia, the acute brain injury is characterized by lesions in the basal ganglia and cortex. A less severe episode of hypoxia may allow initial neurologic recovery followed by the pathologic demyelination characteristic of DPHL. Microscopic examination reveals severe diffuse demyelination with axonal sparing. Reactive astrocytes and macrophages are present, and there is no evidence of intramyelinic vacuolization, thus distinguishing it from heroin inhalation leukoencephalopathy.[4,13]

Although there are many diverse causes of cerebral hypoxia, they are categorized into 4 mechanisms in *Plum and Posner's Diagnosis of Stupor and Coma*[14]: hypoxic hypoxia (low oxygen tension: high altitudes and asphyxial gases), anemic hypoxia (decreased oxygen carrying capacity: anemia and hemoglobinopathy), ischemic hypoxia (insufficient cerebral blood flow: shock, myocardial infarction, and stroke), and histotoxic hypoxia (mitochondrial toxins: cyanide and CO). All 4 mechanisms are equally capable of producing insufficient oxygenation of the brain tissue.[14]

The exact mechanism of the delayed-onset leukoencephalopathy is not yet clear. One theory suggests that hypoxia/hypoperfusion induces necrosis of the oligodendroglia in the border zones between cerebral vascular territories.[15] The delayed onset of symptoms is then due to the time between oligodendroglial injury and loss of myelin.[2] If this were the isolated mechanism, however, DPHL should be much more common. The infrequency of DPHL indicates the possibility of a requisite genetic susceptibility. Some investigators have proposed pseudodeficiency of arylsulfatase A as a predisposing condition[7,13]; however, cases of DPHL with normal arylsulfatase A levels have been reported.[2,15,16] Thus, although pseudodeficiency of arylsulfatase A may predispose to DPHL, it is not a prerequisite condition. There may be other enzyme deficiencies with similar effect or additional undiscovered predisposing conditions.

Heroin use has been associated with DPHL in the setting of associated respiratory depression and hypoxia. Heroin pyrolysate (vapor) likely has additional mechanisms of toxicity and produces a clinical syndrome of "chasing the dragon" leukoencephalopathy that is distinct from DPHL by radiologic and pathologic findings (discussed later).

Treatment and Prognosis

Aggressive supportive care is the core of treatment. No effective pharmaceutical or interventional therapy is known. An unsuccessful trial of immunomodulatory therapy (high-dose steroids and plasmapheresis) has been reported in DPHL after ethanol and morphine intoxication.[17] Otherwise, there are no available data on specific treatment of this condition.

There are limited data on the prognosis of patients who develop DPHL that is not related to CO exposure. Although death has been reported,[17] most patients experience some functional recovery with variable degrees of persistent cognitive and neurologic deficits.[2,4,7,9,13,15,16,18] Neurorehabilitation with multimodality therapies is essential for continued recovery.[10]

Delayed Leukoencephalopathy of Carbon Monoxide Toxicity

The delayed leukoencephalopathy of acute CO toxicity is a subtype of DPHL. There are, however, clinical features and pathologic mechanisms that make this a distinct clinical entity. This is the group of patients with DPHL that are the best defined in the literature. In 1983, Choi published a large case series of 2360 patients with acute CO toxicity.[1] DNS were diagnosed in 65 cases (2.75%) with a mean lucid interval of 22.4 days (range 2–40 days).[1]

Characteristic clinical features of DNS include memory and cognitive deficits, apathy, mutism, urinary incontinence, and gait disturbance. Signs referable to the frontal lobe (primitive reflexes) and basal ganglia (masked facies and rigidity) are common, whereas cerebellar signs are uncommon. Incidence of delayed symptoms seems to increase with the duration of unconsciousness from acute toxicity. The sequelae can occur in patients who had retained consciousness during the acute intoxication, however. In 2 case series with more than 3000 patients with acute CO toxicity, DNS did not occur in any patient under the age of 30 years,[1,19] suggesting an increased susceptibility in older adults.

The MRI findings in delayed leukoencephalopathy after acute CO toxicity are the same as those in DPHL. Acutely, there may be lesions in the basal ganglia on MRI, likely reflective of a more severe event and the susceptibility of the basal ganglia to hypoxia and hypotension induced by cellular asphyxiants. These are usually characterized by T2-sequence hyperintensity that may persist on the MRI done for the delayed symptoms (Fig. 1).[20,21] Single photon-emission CT (SPECT) in patients with DNS reveals diffuse, patchy hypoperfusion throughout the cerebral cortex, and some patients show a correlation between improvement in perfusion and clinical improvement.[22,23]

Although the mechanism of inadequate oxygen supply in DPHL may be any or a combination of the first 3 of *Plum and Posner's* mechanisms (hypoxic, anemic, or ischemic), CO toxicity also causes histotoxic hypoxia.[14] CO causes cellular hypoxia by replacing oxyhemoglobin with carboxyhemoglobin, resulting in a functional anemia, and shifting the oxygen-dissociation curve to the left, resulting in decreased oxygen delivery. This mechanism alone, however, is not sufficient to explain toxicity. In both animal and human studies, the level of carboxyhemoglobin in the blood

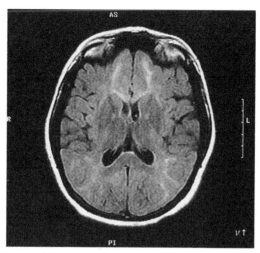

Fig. 1. DPHL in a 46-year-old woman after recovery from acute CO toxicity 3 weeks prior. The bilateral basal ganglia lesions were present on MRI performed on day 3 after acute CO toxicity. The MRI above was performed 6 days after the onset of pseudobulbar affect, confusion, and memory loss. It shows FLAIR hyperintense lesions in the periventricular white matter of both hemispheres.

correlates poorly with the severity of clinical effects.[24,25] CO is a direct cellular toxin via binding to cytochromes, resulting in disruption of oxidative metabolism. It also seems to increase nitric oxide levels leading to oxygen-free radical production. This then may initiate a cascade of events starting with activation of intravascular neutrophils and culminating in brain lipid peroxidation.[26,27]

Treatment of DNS, once it has occurred, is supportive care. Certainly, the standard of care in the setting of acute CO poisoning is high-flow oxygen to treat hypoxia and enhance elimination of CO. There is, however, much debate about the use of hyperbaric oxygen therapy (HBOT) to prevent DNS. To date, 7 prospective randomized controlled trials have compared HBOT with normobaric oxygen for acute CO poisoning.[28–34] Four studies show a benefit of HBOT over normobaric oxygen and 3 do not. Differences in HBOT protocols and outcome measures make definitive conclusions difficult. In general, HBOT is recommended for patients with loss of consciousness, altered mental status, focal neurologic deficits, cardiovascular dysfunction, or severe metabolic acidosis.[35] HBOT is also recommended for pregnant women with CO-hemoglobin levels greater than 15% to 20%, due to the tight binding of CO to fetal hemoglobin. Those patients not meeting these criteria for HBOT should receive normobaric oxygen at 100% by tight-fitting face mask for 6 to 12 hours.[26] The prognosis of DNS is good, with recovery or near-recovery in 61% to 75% of patients within 1 year.[1,19]

HEROIN INHALATION LEUKOENCEPHALOPATHY

The smoking of heroin is a practice that began in Shanghai in the 1920s. "Chasing the dragon" is a method of smoking heroin, born in Hong Kong in the 1950s, that involves inhalation of the vapor (pyrolysate) of heated heroin, typically by using a flame to heat the heroin on folded aluminium foil. Because the hydrochloride form of heroin has become less available over time, it has been replaced by the freebase form. Although the hydrochloride is more easily dissolved in water for injection, the freebase form of heroin is poorly soluble in water but sublimates easily when heated. Thus, chasing the dragon as a technique has become more prevalent because of the availability of the freebase form of heroin as well as the safety concerns surrounding injection methods.[36] The bioavailability of inhaling the vapors of heated heroin is good,[37] especially when in the base form, and may be augmented by the presence of caffeine or barbiturates.[36]

Clinical Features

The first cases of heroin pyrolysate–induced leukoencephalopathy were described by Wolters and colleagues[38] in 1982. The clinical syndrome is characterized by 3 stages, through which each patient may or may not progress. The first stage manifests as a primarily cerebellar syndrome with gait and limb ataxia, soft pseudobulbar speech, apathy, and akathisia. In the second stage, worsening ataxia, spastic paresis, choreoathetoid movements, and myoclonus may occur. Primitive reflexes (palmomental, snout, and oculomandibular) may also emerge in this stage. The terminal stage is characterized by hyperpyrexia, hypotonic paresis, akinetic mutism, and stretching spasms.[38,39] Long and colleagues[40] describe these stretching spasms as "opisthotonic and decerebrate-like posturing."

Progression through these stages occurs over weeks to months.[37,41,42] Of Wolters and colleagues'[38] 47 patients, 26 progressed to the second stage and 11 reached the third, terminal stage. The diagnosis is made on the basis of clinical and imaging features: history of heroin inhalation, cerebellar syndrome, and symmetric white matter lesions of the cerebellum and posterior cerebrum. A recent case series of 27 patients from British Columbia included 1 case of mild symptoms after a single use; all others had used heroin by inhalation for 3 years or more.[42] Some of the cases report the onset of symptoms coinciding with heroin withdrawal,[43,44] whereas others describe onset of symptoms during continued heroin use.[44–48]

Radiologic Findings

The classic findings on MRI include abnormally high T2 signal in symmetric distribution in the cerebellar and posterior cerebral hemispheres, including the posterior limbs of the internal capsule (**Fig. 2**).[39,41,45,49,50] There is relative sparing of the dentate nuclei in the cerebellum, the subcortical U-fibers in the posterior cerebrum, and the anterior limbs of the internal capsules as well as the gray matter in general.[41,46,49] Other reported areas of cerebral involvement include bilateral hippocampi and basal ganglia,[45] thalami,[51] and the corpus callosum.[41,50,52] Reported areas of brainstem

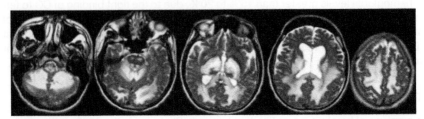

Fig. 2. Chasing the dragon leukoencephalopathy in a 24-year-old man. T2-weighted images of the brain show hyperintense signal in the cerebellum, brainstem, posterior limbs of the internal capsules, thalami, and occipital lobes. (*From* Bartlett E, Mikulis DJ. Chasing "chasing the dragon" with MRI: leukoencephalopathy in drug abuse. Br J Radiol 2005;78:997–1004; with permission.)

involvement include the superior cerebellar peduncles,[38,43] medial lemniscus,[49,50,52] and pyramidal tracts.[49,50,52] Cases that have reported normal signal in the cerebellum either involved intravenous use of heroin or did not establish clear evidence of heroin inhalation.[53–55]

The MRI lesions do not enhance with contrast[39,50] and are typically not diffusion restricted, although diffusion restriction has been reported on MRI performed early in the clinical course when the cellular damage is likely ongoing.[50] Magnetic resonance (MR) spectroscopy demonstrates a reduced N-acetylaspartate peak and an inverted lactate doublet[50,56] with a normal or reduced choline peak.[51] N-acetylaspartate is a marker of neuronal integrity, so the reduction may be secondary to either axonal injury or mitochondrial damage. Choline elevation occurs with demyelination, and the absence of this finding supports the conclusion that demyelination does not occur in this condition. The inverted lactate doublet indicates increased brain lactate content, which suggests conversion to anaerobic metabolism. This constellation of findings on MR spectroscopy is most consistent with mitochondrial dysfunction.[39,41,51,56]

Pathophysiology and Pathologic Findings

Because the classic chasing the dragon leukoencephalopathy does not typically occur with other methods of heroin use, the etiology is most likely related to the method of preparation or a contaminant of the heroin used for inhalation. Triethyltin can be formed from inorganic tin under some conditions and is known to cause a myelinopathy. Tests on commonly available aluminum foil have not demonstrated levels of tin high enough to account for the clinical syndrome.[41] Evaluations of street heroin samples have revealed only known contaminants and cutting agents,[36,42,57,58] none of which is particularly neurotoxic. The rarity of this complication and the occurrence of small epidemics imply that if a contaminant is the cause, it is one added sporadically at the end of the production process.[42] In addition, leukoencephalopathy does not reliably occur in all persons exposed to the same heroin at the same time,[41,47] suggesting the possibility of a required genetic predisposition. Because of the pathologic findings of vacuolar myelinopathy, it is expected that the etiologic toxin is lipophilic[46]; however, the exact cause of this condition remains elusive.

Gross neuropathologic evaluation reveals significant edema. Microscopically, spongiform degeneration of the white matter, characterized by vacuolization within the myelin, is apparent.[59,60] The vacuoles may be so abundant as to coalesce into larger voids.[38] There is reduction in the number of oligodendrocytes without evidence of myelin breakdown products.[59] Axonal degeneration with vacuolar degeneration and mitochondrial swelling may be present as well.[38] Gray matter is unaffected as are the subcortical U-fibers, spinal cord, and peripheral nerves. The pathologic changes usually seen after severe hypoxia, including ischemia-induced neuronal changes and vascular congestion, are notably absent.[40,44,58,59]

Creutzfeldt-Jakob disease is a prion-induced spongiform degeneration that largely affects gray matter. Other causes of spongiform leukoencephalopathy are triethyltin, hexachlorophene, actinomycin D, isonicotinic acid, hydrazine, cycloleucine, cuprizone, and ethidium bromide.[41]

Treatment and Prognosis

The mortality rate in the original case series of 47 patients was 23%.[38] A recent case series of 27 patients reports a mortality rate of 48%.[42] The rarity of this disease process precludes prospective studies to determine risk factors and treatment for heroin pyrolysate-induced spongiform leukoencephalopathy. The features of MR spectroscopy and neuropathology findings support the hypothesis that mitochondrial dysfunction is a contributor to the pathophysiology. Some authors report improvement in symptoms after treatment with an antioxidant drug regimen of ubiquinone (coenzyme Q), vitamin C, and vitamin E.[41,48] Given the favorable side-effect profile of this drug combination, treatment should be considered when the diagnosis is made.

POSTERIOR REVERSIBLE ENCEPHALOPATHY SYNDROME

PRES is a condition with many names. First described as reversible posterior leukoencephalopathy syndrome in 1996, it is a clinicoradiologic diagnosis that is associated with an ever-growing number of medical conditions. It has been called reversible posterior cerebral edema syndrome, hyperperfusion encephalopathy, and brain capillary leak syndrome, but is now commonly titled PRES. Although PRES accurately describes the typical clinical presentation and radiologic findings, some dispute this title because cerebral involvement is not always confined to the territory of the posterior circulation. Severe cases may have areas of cerebral infarction or hemorrhage; thus, the condition is not always reversible. It is perhaps appropriate that it is no longer termed a leukoencephalopathy because the gray matter is often involved, albeit to a lesser extent, and this is frequently manifested by seizures.

In the original case series of 15 patients by Hinchey and colleagues[61] in 1996, 8 were on immunosuppressive therapy, 3 had eclampsia, and 4 had renal disease. Of these patients, 12 had acute hypertension and 11 had seizures. The medical conditions that have a well-established association with PRES are hypertension, eclampsia, autoimmune disease, sepsis/shock, cancer chemotherapy, immunosuppressive therapy, and transplantation.[62] The occurrence of the cerebral vasogenic edema that typifies PRES in this plethora of disease states makes the determination of its pathogenesis complex. This discussion focuses on toxin-induced PRES (ie, immunosuppressive and chemotherapeutic agents).

Clinical Features

The range of clinical symptoms caused by PRES is varied but typically includes headache, encephalopathy, nausea, and vision loss. Signs and symptoms may develop over hours to days. Seizures may occur at the onset of symptoms or later in the course. Moderate-to-severe hypertension is present in 70% to 80% of patients; the remainder have mild hypertension or normal blood pressure.[61,63] Cranial nerve deficits may occur but are rare. The diagnosis of PRES is made by the clinical history, neurologic examination, and neuroimaging. The presence of pre-existing conditions, including pregnancy or recent delivery, acute hypertension, autoimmune conditions, renal disease, or cytotoxic therapy, is supportive of the diagnosis. Differential diagnosis includes ischemic or hemorrhagic stroke, subarachnoid hemorrhage, venous sinus thrombosis, obstructive hydrocephalus, encephalitis, vasculitis, and central demyelination syndromes (acute disseminated encephalomyelitis and central pontine myelinolysis).

The immunosuppressive drugs that are most commonly associated with PRES are the calcineurin inhibitors, cyclosporine and tacrolimus. It has also been reported with bevacizumab, interferon, methotrexate, rituximab, sirolimus, sorafenib, sunitinib, fingolimod, and intravenous immunoglobulin.[61,64–76] The chemotherapeutic agents linked with PRES are cisplatin, cytarabine, doxorubicin, cyclophosphamide, gemcitabine, vincristine, and etoposide.[65,77–82] Drug levels do not seem to correlate with development of PRES, as it has been reported to develop in patients with therapeutic levels of both cyclosporine and tacrolimus.[81,83] The route of administration may also be a factor in the development of PRES. For example, intrathecal administration of methotrexate seems to be associated with a higher incidence of PRES than the intravenous route.[84,85] Fluid overload, mild hypertension, and renal dysfunction are also considered risk factors for the development of PRES.[80]

According to a large case series of 4222 patients, the incidence of PRES after solid-organ transplant is 0.49% (21 cases) without a difference between transplant types.[86] An additional 6 cases were reported outside of the study period for a total of 27 cases, and 7 of these 27 cases presented with an isolated seizure. The remaining 20 patients presented with a combination of headache, encephalopathy, and vision change; 12 of these went on to have a seizure. Blood pressure was normal in 8, mildly elevated in 6, and severely elevated in 13.[86] The timing of onset was more likely to be early (within 2 months of transplant) for liver transplantation and later (1 year or longer after transplant) for kidney transplantation. There are few data on the incidence of PRES with specific drugs, although small case series have reported a 1.6% incidence of tacrolimus-associated PRES and a 7.5% incidence of cyclosporin A–associated PRES in hematopoietic stem cell transplant patients.[87,88]

Radiologic Findings

Neuroimaging typically reveals evidence of white matter edema with symmetric involvement of the occipitoparietal regions (**Fig. 3**).[61,63,89,90] Although vasogenic edema is the hallmark of PRES, cases with areas of cytotoxic edema suggestive of focal infarction have been described.[91–93] Thus, although CT usually depicts hypodense lesions in the affected regions, MRI is the diagnostic test of choice because of the utility of diffusion-weighted imaging (DWI) in differentiating vasogenic from cytotoxic edema. Identification of the affected cortical and subcortical areas is best performed by the fluid-attenuated inversion recovery (FLAIR) sequence.[94] Then, DWI and apparent diffusion coefficient (ADC) mapping allow assessment of the type of edema: vasogenic (isointense or hyperintense on DWI and hyperintense on ADC) versus cytotoxic (hyperintense on DWI and hypointense on ADC).[92,93,95]

The classic pattern of involvement in PRES is bilateral and symmetric lesions in the cortex and subcortical white matter of the occipital and parietal lobes. Lesions in the posterior frontal and temporal lobes as well as the cerebellum, brainstem, thalamus, and basal ganglia are increasingly reported.[91] An MRI pattern involving these areas has been termed, atypical PRES, but is likely more common than previously recognized. Although there may be lesions in areas not supplied by the posterior circulation, the predominant MRI findings are posterior. Serial imaging demonstrates improvement or resolution in most cases.

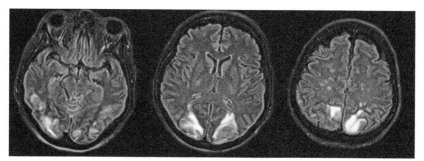

Fig. 3. PRES in a 54-year-old woman who presented with altered mental status, seizures, and vision changes while taking tacrolimus for immunosuppression after liver transplantation. FLAIR images show hyperintensity in the bilateral occipital lobes. She clinically improved after immunosuppression was changed from tacrolimus to cyclosporine.

MR angiography demonstrates findings of diffuse vasoconstriction or focal vaso-constriction alternating with vasodilation, consistent with vasospasm.[96–101] Catheter angiography in patients with PRES reveals similar findings.[99,102–106] Single-photon emission CT (SPECT) results have been less consistent in that some studies have reported hyperperfusion on SPECT and some have reported hypoperfusion.[90,107–109]

Pathophysiology and Pathologic Findings

The origin of PRES is complex and controversial. Vasogenic edema in the subcortical white matter of the posterior circulation, with variable involvement of the cortex and the territory of the anterior circulation, is the accepted cause of symptoms. It is the etiology of the edema that is currently under debate. The hyperperfusion theory holds that abnormal autoregulation allows for increased perfusion in the setting of hypertension, resulting in breakdown of the blood-brain barrier and vasogenic edema.[61,80,90] The relatively reduced number of adrenergic nerves in the vertebrobasilar circulation may predispose this region to the development of edema.[110,111] Alternatively, vasoconstriction, as a normal autoregulatory response to hypertension, leads to hypoperfusion followed by ischemia and vasogenic edema.[112] Endothelial dysfunction, whether from an immunologic process or direct drug toxicity, likely plays a role in pathogenesis as well.[61,75,112]

During the acute phase, pathologic findings on microscopy are consistent with vasogenic edema. Reactive astrocytes with macrophages and lymphocytes have been observed, usually without evidence of inflammation or neuronal damage.[83,113–115] Histopathologic findings on autopsy specimen after a prolonged course demonstrate necrotic foci and other features consistent with ischemia.[81–83,116]

Treatment and Prognosis

Diagnosis of PRES is the initial step in treatment because recognition of the pathologic process leads to identification of etiologic factors. Removal of causative agents, treatment of seizures, and measured lowering of blood pressure are the mainstay of treatment. Transplant patients who require immunosuppression may improve with transition to another immunosuppressive agent or a decrease in the dose.[62] Prognosis is usually good, with recovery over the course of days, after appropriate care is initiated.[61] Delay in diagnosis can result in progression of the edema and may contribute to permanent neurologic sequelae from cerebral infarction or hemorrhage.[95,96] Death is a rarely reported complication.[116,117]

SUMMARY

Leukoencephalopathy is a clinical and radiologic diagnosis with a wide variety of causes, including infections, autoimmune disease, neoplasms, and metabolic disorders as well as many toxins not addressed in this article (eg, radiation, ethanol, and toluene).

DPHL is characterized by recovery from a recent hypoxic event followed by acute onset of neuropsychiatric symptoms. MRI findings include T2-sequence hyperintense lesions in the periventricular white matter of both hemispheres, usually involving the frontal lobes and sparing the cerebellum and brainstem. Treatment is supportive care.

Heroin inhalation leukoencephalopathy usually presents as a cerebellar syndrome in the setting of chronic inhalation of heroin vapor (chasing the dragon). MRI findings include symmetric T2-sequence hyperintense lesions in the cerebellum and posterior cerebral hemispheres. Pathologic evaluation demonstrates intramyelinic vacuolization. Treatment is largely supportive care, although antioxidant therapy may be considered.

PRES is characterized by headache, vision changes, seizures, and alteration of mental status. This may occur in the setting of acute hypertension, eclampsia, autoimmune disease, sepsis/shock, cancer chemotherapy, immunosuppressive therapy, and transplantation. MRI findings include T2-sequence hyperintense lesions in the occipitoparietal regions. Removal of causative medications as well as the treatment of seizures and hypertension is the appropriate treatment regimen.

REFERENCES

1. Choi IS. Delayed neurologic sequelae in carbon monoxide intoxication. Arch Neurol 1983;40:433–5.
2. Lee HB, Lyketsos CG. Delayed post-hypoxic leukoencephalopathy. Psychosomatics 2001;42:530–3.
3. Custodio CM, Basford JR. Delayed postanoxic encephalopathy: a case report and literature review. Arch Phys Med Rehabil 2004;85:502–5.
4. Plum F, Posner JB, Hain RF. Delayed neurological deterioration after anoxia. Arch Intern Med 1962;110:18–25.
5. Hori A, Hirose G, Kataoka S, et al. Delayed postanoxic encephalopathy after strangulation. Serial neuroradiological and neurochemical studies. Arch Neurol 1991;48:871–4.
6. Mizutani T, Shiozawa R, Takemori S, et al. Delayed post-anoxic encephalopathy without relation to carbon monoxide poisoning. Intern Med 1993;32:430–3.
7. Weinberger LM, Schmidley JW, Schafer IA, et al. Delayed postanoxic demyelination and arylsulfatase-A pseudodeficiency. Neurology 1994;44:152–4.
8. Protass LM. Delayed postanoxic encephalopathy after heroin use. Ann Intern Med 1971;74:738–9.
9. Barnett MH, Miller LA, Reddel SW, et al. Reversible delayed leukoencephalopathy following intravenous heroin overdose. J Clin Neurosci 2001;8:165–7.
10. Shprecher D, Mehta L. The syndrome of delayed post-hypoxic leukoencephalopathy. NeuroRehabilitation 2010;26:65–72.
11. Lee MS, Marsden CD. Neurological sequelae following carbon monoxide poisoning clinical course and outcome according to the clinical types and brain computed tomography scan findings. Mov Disord 1994;9:550–8.
12. Chen-Plotkin AS, Pau KT, Schmahmann JD. Delayed leukoencephalopathy after hypoxic-ischemic injury. Arch Neurol 2008;65:144–5.
13. Gottfried JA, Mayer SA, Shungu DC, et al. Delayed posthypoxic demyelination. Association with arylsulfatase A deficiency and lactic acidosis on proton MR spectroscopy. Neurology 1997;49:1400–4.
14. Posner JB, Saper CB, Schiff ND, et al. Plum and Posner's diagnosis of stupor and coma. 4th edition. New York: Oxford University Press; 2007. p. 210–1.
15. Heckmann JG, Erbguth F, Neundörfer B. Delayed postanoxic demyelination registry. Neurology 1998;51:1235–6.
16. Shprecher DR, Flanigan KM, Smith AG, et al. Clinical and diagnostic features of delayed hypoxic leukoencephalopathy. J Neuropsychiatry Clin Neurosci 2008; 20:473–7.
17. Khot S, Walker M, Lacy JM, et al. An unsuccessful trial of immunomodulatory therapy in delayed posthypoxic demyelination. Neurocrit Care 2007;7:253–6.
18. Molloy S, Soh C, Williams TL. Reversible delayed posthypoxic leukoencephalopathy. AJNR Am J Neuroradiol 2006;27:1763–5.
19. Min SK. A brain syndrome associated with delayed neuropsychiatric sequelae following acute carbon monoxide intoxication. Acta Psychiatr Scand 1986;73:80–6.

20. Kawada N, Ochiai N, Kuzuhara S. Diffusion MRI in acute carbon monoxide poisoning. Intern Med 2004;43:639–40.
21. Singhal AB, Topcuoglu MA, Koroshetz WJ. Diffusion MRI in three types of anoxic encephalopathy. J Neurol Sci 2002;196:37–40.
22. Choi IS, Lee MS, Lee YJ, et al. Technetium-99m HM-PAO SPECT in patients with delayed neurologic sequelae after carbon monoxide poisoning. J Korean Med Sci 1992;7:11–8.
23. Choi IS, Kim SK, Lee SS, et al. Evaluation of outcome of delayed neurologic sequelae after carbon monoxide poisoning by technetium-99m hexamethylpropylene amine oxime brain single photon emission computed tomography. Eur Neurol 1995;35:137–42.
24. Norkool DM, Kirkpatrick JN. Treatment of acute carbon monoxide poisoning with hyperbaric oxygen: a review of 115 cases. Ann Emerg Med 1985;14:1168–71.
25. Myers RA. Carbon monoxide poisoning. J Emerg Med 1984;1:245–8.
26. Kao LW, Nañagas KA. Carbon monoxide poisoning. Emerg Med Clin North Am 2004;22:985–1018.
27. Thom SR, Bhopale VM, Han ST, et al. Intravascular neutrophil activation due to carbon monoxide poisoning. Am J Respir Crit Care Med 2006;174:1239–48.
28. Raphael JC, Elkharrat D, Jars-Guincestre MC, et al. Trial of normobaric and hyperbaric oxygen for acute carbon monoxide intoxication. Lancet 1989;2:414–9.
29. Ducassé JL, Celsis P, Marc-Vergnes JP. Non-comatose patients with acute carbon monoxide poisoning: hyperbaric or normobaric oxygenation? Undersea Hyperb Med 1995;22:9–15.
30. Thom SR, Taber RL, Mendiguren II, et al. Delayed neuropsychologic sequelae after carbon monoxide poisoning: prevention by treatment with hyperbaric oxygen. Ann Emerg Med 1995;25:474–80.
31. Mathieu D, Wattel F, Mathieu-Nolf M, et al. Randomized prospective study comparing the effect of HBO versus 12 hours NBO in non-comatose CO poisoned patients: results of interim analysis [abstract]. Undersea Hyperb Med 1996;23:7–8.
32. Scheinkestel CD, Bailey M, Myles PS, et al. Hyperbaric or normobaric oxygen for acute carbon monoxide poisoning: a randomised controlled clinical trial. Med J Aust 1999;170:203–10.
33. Weaver LK, Hopkins RO, Chan KJ, et al. Hyperbaric oxygen for acute carbon monoxide poisoning. N Engl J Med 2002;347:1057–67.
34. Annane D, Chadda K, Gajdos P, et al. Hyperbaric oxygen therapy for acute domestic carbon monoxide poisoning: two randomized controlled trials. Intensive Care Med 2011;37:486–92.
35. Hampson NB, Mathieu D, Piantadosi CA, et al. Carbon monoxide poisoning: interpretation of randomized clinical trials and unresolved treatment issues. Undersea Hyperb Med 2001;28:157–64.
36. Strang J, Griffiths P, Gossop M. Heroin smoking by 'chasing the dragon': origins and history. Addiction 1997;92:673–83 [discussion: 685–95].
37. Hendriks VM, van den Brink W, Blanken P, et al. Heroin self-administration by means of 'chasing the dragon': pharmacodynamics and bioavailability of inhaled heroin. Eur Neuropsychopharmacol 2001;11:241–52.
38. Wolters EC, van Wijngaarden GK, Stam FC, et al. Leucoencephalopathy after inhaling "heroin" pyrolysate. Lancet 1982;2:1233–7.
39. Offiah C, Hall E. Heroin-induced leukoencephalopathy: characterization using MRI, diffusion-weighted imaging, and MR spectroscopy. Clin Radiol 2008;63:146–52.

40. Long H, Deore K, Hoffman RS, et al. A fatal case of spongiform leukoencephalopathy linked to "chasing the dragon". J Toxicol Clin Toxicol 2003;41:887–91.
41. Kriegstein AR, Shungu DC, Millar WS, et al. Leukoencephalopathy and raised brain lactate from heroin vapor inhalation ("chasing the dragon"). Neurology 1999;53:1765–73.
42. Buxton JA, Sebastian R, Clearsky L, et al. Chasing the dragon- Characterizing cases of leukoencephalopathy associated with heroin inhalation in British Columbia. Harm Reduct J 2011;8:3.
43. Weber W, Henkes H, Möller P, et al. Toxic spongiform leucoencephalopathy after inhaling heroin vapour. Eur Radiol 1998;8:749–55.
44. Kriegstein AR, Armitage BA, Kim PY. Heroin inhalation and progressive spongiform leukoencephalopathy. N Engl J Med 1997;336:589–90.
45. Gupta PK, Krishnan PR, Sudhakar PJ. Hippocampal involvement due to heroin inhalation–"chasing the dragon". Clin Neurol Neurosurg 2009;111:278–81.
46. Tan TP, Algra PR, Valk J, et al. Toxic leukoencephalopathy after inhalation of poisoned heroin: MR findings. AJNR Am J Neuroradiol 1994;15:175–8.
47. Celius EG, Andersson S. Leucoencephalopathy after inhalation of heroin: a case report. J Neurol Neurosurg Psychiatry 1996;60:694–5.
48. Gacouin A, Lavoue S, Signouret T, et al. Reversible spongiform leucoencephalopathy after inhalation of heated heroin. Intensive Care Med 2003;29:1012–5.
49. Keogh CF, Andrews GT, Spacey SD, et al. Neuroimaging features of heroin inhalation toxicity: "chasing the dragon". AJR Am J Roentgenol 2003;180:847–50.
50. Hagel J, Andrews G, Vertinsky T, et al. "Chasing the dragon"—imaging of heroin inhalation leukoencephalopathy. Can Assoc Radiol J 2005;56:199–203.
51. Bartlett E, Mikulis DJ. Chasing "chasing the dragon" with MRI: leukoencephalopathy in drug abuse. Br J Radiol 2005;78:997–1004.
52. Au-Yeung K, Lai C. Toxic leucoencephalopathy after heroin inhalation. Australas Radiol 2002;46:306–8.
53. Ryan A, Molloy FM, Farrell MA, et al. Fatal toxic leukoencephalopathy: clinical, radiological, and necropsy findings in two patients. J Neurol Neurosurg Psychiatry 2005;76:1014–6.
54. Chen CY, Lee KW, Lee CC, et al. Heroin-induced spongiform leukoencephalopathy: value of diffusion MR imaging. J Comput Assist Tomogr 2000;24:735–7.
55. Maschke M, Fehlings T, Kastrup O, et al. Toxic leukoencephalopathy after intravenous consumption of heroin and cocaine with unexpected clinical recovery. J Neurol 1999;246:850–1.
56. Chang WC, Lo CP, Kao HW, et al. MRI features of spongiform leukoencephalopathy following heroin inhalation. Neurology 2006;67:504.
57. Brenneisen R, Hasler F. GC/MS determination of pyrolysis products from diacetylmorphine and adulterants of street heroin samples. J Forensic Sci 2002;47:885–8.
58. Sempere AP, Posada I, Ramo C, et al. Spongiform leucoencephalopathy after inhaling heroin. Lancet 1991;338:320.
59. Büttner A, Mall G, Penning R, et al. The neuropathology of heroin abuse. Forensic Sci Int 2000;113:435–42.
60. Halloran O, Ifthikharuddin S, Samkoff L. Leukoencephalopathy from "chasing the dragon". Neurology 2005;64:1755.
61. Hinchey J, Chaves C, Appignani B, et al. A reversible posterior leukoencephalopathy syndrome. N Engl J Med 1996;334:494–500.
62. Bartynski WS. Posterior reversible encephalopathy syndrome, part 1: fundamental imaging and clinical features. AJNR Am J Neuroradiol 2008;29:1036–42.

63. Mukherjee P, McKinstry RC. Reversible posterior leukoencephalopathy syndrome: evaluation with diffusion-tensor MR imaging. Radiology 2001;219: 756–65.

64. Glusker P, Recht L, Lane B. Reversible posterior leukoencephalopathy syndrome and bevacizumab. N Engl J Med 2006;354:980–2 [discussion: 980–2].

65. Incecik F, Hergüner MO, Altunbasak S, et al. Evaluation of nine children with reversible posterior encephalopathy syndrome. Neurol India 2009;57:475–8.

66. Dicuonzo F, Salvati A, Palma M, et al. Posterior reversible encephalopathy syndrome associated with methotrexate neurotoxicity: conventional magnetic resonance and diffusion-weighted imaging findings. J Child Neurol 2009;24: 1013–8.

67. Mavragani CP, Vlachoyiannopoulos PG, Kosmas N, et al. A case of reversible posterior leucoencephalopathy syndrome after rituximab infusion. Rheumatology 2004;43:1450–1.

68. Moskowitz A, Nolan C, Lis E, et al. Posterior reversible encephalopathy syndrome due to sirolimus. Bone Marrow Transplant 2007;39:653–4.

69. Govindarajan R, Adusumilli J, Baxter DL, et al. Reversible posterior leukoencephalopathy syndrome induced by RAF kinase inhibitor BAY 43-9006. J Clin Oncol 2006;24:e48.

70. Cumurciuc R, Martinez-Almoyna L, Henry C, et al. Posterior reversible encephalopathy syndrome during sunitinib therapy. Rev Neurol (Paris) 2008;164:605–7.

71. Kappos L, Antel J, Comi G, et al. Oral fingolimod (FTY720) for relapsing multiple sclerosis. N Engl J Med 2006;355:1124–40.

72. Koichihara R, Hamano SI, Yamashita S, et al. Posterior reversible encephalopathy syndrome associated with IVIG in a patient with Guillain-Barré syndrome. Pediatr Neurol 2008;39:123–5.

73. Belmouaz S, Desport E, Leroy F, et al. Posterior reversible encephalopathy induced by intravenous immunoglobulin. Nephrol Dial Transplant 2008;23:417–9.

74. De Klippel N, Sennesael J, Lamote J, et al. Cyclosporin leukoencephalopathy induced by intravenous lipid solution. Lancet 1992;339:1114.

75. Wu Q, Marescaux C, Wolff V, et al. Tacrolimus-associated posterior reversible encephalopathy syndrome after solid organ transplantation. Eur Neurol 2010; 64:169–77.

76. Bodkin CL, Eidelman BH. Sirolimus-induced posterior reversible encephalopathy. Neurology 2007;68:2039–40.

77. Ito Y, Arahata Y, Goto Y, et al. Cisplatin neurotoxicity presenting as reversible posterior leukoencephalopathy syndrome. AJNR Am J Neuroradiol 1998;19:415–7.

78. Hemmaway C, Mian A, Nagy Z. Images in haematology. Irreversible blindness secondary to posterior reversible encephalopathy syndrome following CHOP combination chemotherapy. Br J Haematol 2010;150:129.

79. Russell MT, Nassif AS, Cacayorin ED, et al. Gemcitabine-associated posterior reversible encephalopathy syndrome: MR imaging and MR spectroscopy findings. Magn Reson Imaging 2001;19:129–32.

80. Tam CS, Galanos J, Seymour JF, et al. Reversible posterior leukoencephalopathy syndrome complicating cytotoxic chemotherapy for hematologic malignancies. Am J Hematol 2004;77:72–6.

81. Reece DE, Frei-Lahr DA, Shepherd JD, et al. Neurologic complications in allogeneic bone marrow transplant patients receiving cyclosporin. Bone Marrow Transplant 1991;8:393–401.

82. Vaughn DJ, Jarvik JG, Hackney D, et al. High-dose cytarabine neurotoxicity: MR findings during the acute phase. AJNR Am J Neuroradiol 1993;14:1014–6.

83. Bartynski WS, Zeigler Z, Spearman MP, et al. Etiology of cortical and white matter lesions in cyclosporin-A and FK-506 neurotoxicity. AJNR Am J Neuroradiol 2001; 22:1901–14.

84. Mahoney DH Jr, Shuster JJ, Nitschke R, et al. Acute neurotoxicity in children with B-precursor acute lymphoid leukemia: an association with intermediate-dose intravenous methotrexate and intrathecal triple therapy–a Pediatric Oncology Group study. J Clin Oncol 1998;16:1712–22.

85. Asato R, Akiyama Y, Ito M, et al. Nuclear magnetic resonance abnormalities of the cerebral white matter in children with acute lymphoblastic leukemia and malignant lymphoma during and after central nervous system prophylactic treatment with intrathecal methotrexate. Cancer 1992;70:1997–2004.

86. Bartynski WS, Tan HP, Boardman JF, et al. Posterior reversible encephalopathy syndrome after solid organ transplantation. AJNR Am J Neuroradiol 2008;29: 924–30.

87. Wong R, Beguelin GZ, de Lima M, et al. Tacrolimus-associated posterior reversible encephalopathy syndrome after allogeneic haematopoietic stem cell transplantation. Br J Haematol 2003;122:128–34.

88. Noè A, Cappelli B, Biffi A, et al. High incidence of severe cyclosporine neurotoxicity in children affected by haemoglobinopaties undergoing myeloablative haematopoietic stem cell transplantation: early diagnosis and prompt intervention ameliorates neurological outcome. Ital J Pediatr 2010;36:14.

89. Duncan R, Hadley D, Bone I, et al. Blindness in eclampsia: CT and MR imaging. J Neurol Neurosurg Psychiatry 1989;52:899–902.

90. Schwartz RB, Jones KM, Kalina P, et al. Hypertensive encephalopathy: findings on CT, MR imaging, and SPECT imaging in 14 cases. AJR Am J Roentgenol 1992;159:379–83.

91. McKinney AM, Short J, Truwit CL, et al. Posterior reversible encephalopathy syndrome: incidence of atypical regions of involvement and imaging findings. AJR Am J Roentgenol 2007;189:904–12.

92. Donmez FY, Basaran C, Kayahan Ulu EM, et al. MRI features of posterior reversible encephalopathy syndrome in 33 patients. J Neuroimaging 2010;20:22–8.

93. Finocchi V, Bozzao A, Bonamini M, et al. Magnetic resonance imaging in posterior reversible encephalopathy syndrome: report of three cases and review of literature. Arch Gynecol Obstet 2005;271:79–85.

94. Casey SO, Sampaio RC, Michel E, et al. Posterior reversible encephalopathy syndrome: utility of fluid-attenuated inversion recovery MR imaging in the detection of cortical and subcortical lesions. AJNR Am J Neuroradiol 2000;21:1199–206.

95. Ay H, Buonanno FS, Schaefer PW, et al. Posterior leukoencephalopathy without severe hypertension: utility of diffusion-weighted MRI. Neurology 1998;51:1369–76.

96. Henderson RD, Rajah T, Nicol AJ, et al. Posterior leukoencephalopathy following intrathecal chemotherapy with MRA-documented vasospasm. Neurology 2003; 60:326–8.

97. Thaipisuttikul I, Phanthumchinda K. Recurrent reversible posterior leukoencephalopathy in a patient with systemic lupus erythematosus. J Neurol 2005; 252:230–1.

98. Sweany JM, Bartynski WS, Boardman JF. "Recurrent" posterior reversible encephalopathy syndrome: report of 3 cases–PRES can strike twice! J Comput Assist Tomogr 2007;31:148–56.

99. Bartynski WS, Boardman JF. Catheter angiography, MR angiography, and MR perfusion in posterior reversible encephalopathy syndrome. AJNR Am J Neuroradiol 2008;29:447–55.

100. Ito T, Sakai T, Inagawa S, et al. MR angiography of cerebral vasospasm in pre-eclampsia. AJNR Am J Neuroradiol 1995;16:1344–6.
101. Lin JT, Wang SJ, Fuh JL, et al. Prolonged reversible vasospasm in cyclosporin A-induced encephalopathy. AJNR Am J Neuroradiol 2003;24:102–4.
102. Ito Y, Niwa H, Iida T, et al. Post-transfusion reversible posterior leukoencephalopathy syndrome with cerebral vasoconstriction. Neurology 1997;49:1174–5.
103. Trommer BL, Homer D, Mikhael MA. Cerebral vasospasm and eclampsia. Stroke 1988;19:326–9.
104. Bartynski WS, Sanghvi A. Neuroimaging of delayed eclampsia. Report of 3 cases and review of the literature. J Comput Assist Tomogr 2003;27:699–713.
105. Aeby A, David P, Fricx C, et al. Posterior reversible encephalopathy syndrome revealing acute post-streptococcal glomerulonephritis. J Child Neurol 2006; 21:250–1.
106. Geraghty JJ, Hoch DB, Robert ME, et al. Fatal puerperal cerebral vasospasm and stroke in a young woman. Neurology 1991;41:1145–7.
107. Apollon KM, Robinson JN, Schwartz RB, et al. Cortical blindness in severe pre-eclampsia: computed tomography, magnetic resonance imaging, and single-photon-emission computed tomography findings. Obstet Gynecol 2000;95: 1017–9.
108. Sanchez-Carpintero R, Narbona J, López de Mesa R, et al. Transient posterior encephalopathy induced by chemotherapy in children. Pediatr Neurol 2001; 24:145–8.
109. Naidu K, Moodley J, Corr P, et al. Single photon emission and cerebral compu-terised tomographic scan and transcranial Doppler sonographic findings in eclampsia. Br J Obstet Gynaecol 1997;104:1165–72.
110. Edvinsson L, Owman C, Sjöberg NO. Autonomic nerves, mast cells, and amine receptors in human brain vessels. A histochemical and pharmacological study. Brain Res 1976;115:377–93.
111. Beausang-Linder M, Bill A. Cerebral circulation in acute arterial hypertension—protective effects of sympathetic nervous activity. Acta Physiol Scand 1981;111: 193–9.
112. Bartynski WS. Posterior reversible encephalopathy syndrome, part 2: contro-versies surrounding pathophysiology of vasogenic edema. AJNR Am J Neuro-radiol 2008;29:1043–9.
113. Lanzino G, Cloft H, Hemstreet MK, et al. Reversible posterior leukoencephalop-athy following organ transplantation. Description of two cases. Clin Neurol Neu-rosurg 1997;99:222–6.
114. Thyagarajan GK, Cobanoglu A, Johnston W. FK506-induced fulminant leukoen-cephalopathy after single-lung transplantation. Ann Thorac Surg 1997;64(14): 61–4.
115. Schiff D, Lopes MB. Neuropathological correlates of reversible posterior leu-koencephalopathy. Neurocrit Care 2005;2:303–5.
116. Greenwood MJ, Dodds AJ, Garricik R, et al. Posterior leukoencephalopathy in association with the tumour lysis syndrome in acute lymphoblastic leukaemia—a case with clinicopathological correlation. Leuk Lymphoma 2003;44:719–21.
117. Cain MS, Burton GV, Holcombe RF. Fatal leukoencephalopathy in a patient with non-Hodgkin's lymphoma treated with CHOP chemotherapy and high-dose steroids. Am J Med Sci 1998;315:202–7.

Toluene Abuse and White Matter
A Model of Toxic Leukoencephalopathy

Christopher M. Filley, MD

KEYWORDS

- Toluene • White matter • Dementia • Toxic • Leukoencephalopathy • Inhalants

KEY POINTS

- Toluene is rapidly absorbed through the lungs after inhalation and quickly crosses the blood–brain barrier to reach the lipid-rich central nervous system, sparing the peripheral nervous system.
- The management of toluene and other inhalant abuse involves an understanding of both the prognosis of those who are affected and the treatment of this form of substance abuse.
- From a research perspective, toluene abuse offers an instructive model of toxic leukoencephalopathy.

Of the many substances of abuse that can result in serious medical consequences, inhalants are among the least well recognized.[1] Commonly inhaled in large quantities for their euphorigenic effects, inhalants include a wide range of volatile chemicals that may be sought out as abusable substances. Hundreds of agents can be inhaled, adding to the difficulty of establishing organizing principles within this field; some of the more commonly abused inhalants are shown in **Table 1**. In contrast to many other abusable substances that receive more publicity and medical attention, inhalants are typically inexpensive, readily available, and legal, so that few barriers exist to their consumption. While the effects of acute intoxication can be dramatic, the lasting adverse effects of inhalants may also be highly injurious, and many forms of nervous system toxicity are among the most notable sequelae of the chronic abuse of inhalants. In particular, the brain is the primary target of toluene (methylbenzene), the major solvent in spray paint and a constituent of many other easily obtained commercial and industrial products. Advances in understanding of the specific effects of toluene on the brain have helped considerably to clarify the neurotoxicity of inhalant abuse.

Over the last 30 years, a substantial literature has been developed that describes the effects of toluene on the white matter of the brain. This disorder, termed toluene

Behavioral Neurology Section, University of Colorado School of Medicine, 12631 East 17th Avenue, MS B185, Aurora, CO 80045, USA
E-mail address: christopher.filley@ucdenver.edu

Psychiatr Clin N Am 36 (2013) 293–302
http://dx.doi.org/10.1016/j.psc.2013.02.008
0193-953X/13/$ – see front matter © 2013 Elsevier Inc. All rights reserved.

Table 1
Some commonly abused inhalants

Inhalant	Source(s)
Toluene	Spray paint, glues, cements, paint remover, paint thinner, gasoline
Xylene	Spray paint, glues, cements, gasoline
Hexane	Gasoline, glues, cements
Methyl chloride	Glues, cements
Methyl ethyl ketone	Glues, cements
Methyl butyl ketone	Glues, cements
Benzene	Gasoline, glues, cements
Trichloroethylene	Dry cleaning fluids, degreasers, correction fluid, glues, cements
Tetrachloroethylene	Dry cleaning fluids, degreasers, spot remover, glues
Trichloroethane	Dry cleaning fluids, degreasers, correction fluid, spot remover
Methylene chloride	Paint remover, lacquer thinner
Methanol	Paint remover, lacquer thinner
Petroleum distillates	Paint thinner, spot remover
Butane	Lighter fluid, hair spray, deodorant, spray paint
Propane	Lighter fluid, hair spray, deodorant, spray paint
Nitrous oxide	Food product propellant, gaseous anesthetic

leukoencephalopathy, produces a variety of neurologic disturbances, the most prominent of which is dementia. In light of these findings, this article has 2 objectives:

1. The problem of toluene abuse will be considered as an instructive example of this relatively neglected area of substance abuse.
2. The effects of toluene on the brain white matter will be discussed as a model of the broader topic of toxic leukoencephalopathy,[2] other examples of which are considered elsewhere in this issue.

To begin, a brief review of the neurobiology of brain white matter will be useful.

WHITE MATTER NEUROBIOLOGY
Anatomy

White matter comprises about half the volume of the adult brain,[3] and roughly 135,000 km of myelinated fibers course within the cerebrum.[4] Macroscopically, white matter consists of millions of myelinated axons that are closely adjacent within tracts, fascicles, bundles, and peduncles; in the brain, neuroanatomists have long distinguished between projection, association, and commissural fiber systems.[5] Association and commissural tracts are most critical for neurobehavioral function, as they link cortical and subcortical gray matter regions into neural networks.[6,7] Also important are smaller white matter fascicles that are found within the cerebral cortex and deep gray matter of the basal ganglia, thalamus, and cerebellum.[8] White matter neuroanatomy is highly complex, and much remains unknown; modern neuroimaging is adding new information that supplements the findings of classic neuroanatomy, and finer details of cerebral macroconnectivity are becoming more clear.[9] The microscopic structure of white matter features myelin, a mixture of 70% lipid and 30% protein that encircles many axons except for unmyelinated zones called nodes of Ranvier, and oligodendrocytes, glial cells of the central nervous system (CNS) responsible for myelin formation.[10,11]

Physiology

The defining functional characteristic of white matter is the increase of axonal conduction velocity conferred by the presence of myelin. By virtue of saltatory conduction enabled by the nodes of Ranvier, myelinated axons conduct action potentials much more rapidly than unmyelinated fibers, and the efficiency of widely distributed neural networks is thus greatly enhanced.[10] The assumption that slowed neural transmission manifests as slowed cognition is in fact proving to be correct; much recent evidence indicates that processing speed is indeed dependent on the integrity of white matter tracts,[12,13] supporting the notion that the transfer of information within the brain is facilitated by myelinated systems. This capacity of white matter permits the highly integrated operations of large-scale neural networks distributed within and between the hemispheres, seamlessly linking the gray matter of the cerebral cortex with other cortical regions and many subcortical nuclei.[14] Distributed neural networks are conceptualized as subserving arousal, attention, executive function, memory, language, praxis, visuospatial ability, recognition, and a variety of emotional domains including motivation, comportment, social cognition, and others that are steadily being better defined.[14,15] In all of these networks, the distinction can be maintained between the microconnectivity of gray matter, in which synaptic function subserves information processing, and the macroconnectivity of white matter, whereby widely dispersed gray matter areas are unified into functionally related neural ensembles.[14,15]

INHALANT ABUSE

The intentional inhalation of volatile substances is a worldwide phenomenon that appears most often in adolescents and young adults with disadvantaged socioeconomic background, higher rates of mental illness, and frequent involvement with the criminal justice system.[1] In the United States, reported prevalence figures of inhalant use have been startlingly high. It has been reported that 19.9% of eighth graders have tried inhalants at least once, with particularly high prevalence noted among Hispanics and Native Americans.[16] A more recent review reports that an estimated 9% of the US population over age 12, some 22.5 million people, have used inhalants at least once with psychoactive intent.[1] Fortunately, many individuals quickly abandon the practice, and inhalant abuse is thought be considerably less common than inhalant use. However, as many as 50% of inhalant users may be at risk for inhalant abuse,[1] indicating that this problem clearly merits attention as a medical and social challenge.

Inhalants remain the least studied class of psychoactive chemicals,[1] but their propensity for harm is significant. While undue alarm over most incidental or casual exposure to inhalants is unwarranted, the medical consequences of inhalant abuse can involve many organ systems and a wide range of severity, from mild and fully reversible syndromes to severe disability and death.[1,16] The neurologic effects associated with the period of intoxication can include headache, dizziness, incoordination, and mental status alterations ranging from acute confusional state to coma, and a host of chronic deficits that will be described. In addition, cardiac (arrythmias), pulmonary (bronchitis), renal (renal tubular acidosis), hepatic (elevated liver function enzymes), hematologic (bone marrow suppression), immune (reduced cellular immunity), and teratogenic (fetal solvent syndrome) effects have all been noted.[1,16]

One of the issues facing investigators seeking to understand the effects of inhalants is the problem of multiple or mixed inhalant abuse, which extends to the dilemma of multidrug abuse as a more general phenomenon. People who are exposed to more than 1 solvent or abusable drug necessarily have more than potential toxic exposure, and detecting the specific effects of 1 toxin is challenging. This issue also impacts the investigation of solvent exposure in the workplace, which, while far less extensive than in inhalant abusers, still requires a secure determination of which solvent produces which specific effects. In this regard, the study of toluene abuse has special importance, as reviewed studies have made deliberate efforts to identify individuals whose inhalant abuse is generally limited to 1 agent. Toluene is the solvent that has yielded the most useful data elucidating long-term neurologic and neurobehavioral consequences.

WHITE MATTER DEMENTIA FROM TOLUENE LEUKOENCEPHALOPATHY

Toluene is rapidly absorbed through the lungs after inhalation and quickly crosses the blood–brain barrier to reach the lipid-rich CNS, sparing the peripheral nervous system. The principle site of action of toluene is known to be the brain, and the chronic neurologic effects of high concentrations of toluene in abusers of this solvent have been steadily documented (**Table 2**).[17–23] An important point is that abusers must be studied during periods of abstinence so that lasting toxic effects can be distinguished from the acute effects, which are typically reversible.[18] Persistent neurologic impairment from toluene sniffing in individuals studied during abstinence was first reported in 1961 with observations of cerebellar involvement,[17] but the advent of magnetic resonance imaging (MRI) in the early 1980s led to the recognition that the major neurologic sequel of toluene abuse is dementia. MRI facilitates the identification of many previously obscure or undetectable brain lesions, and in this era, the first observations were made of the specific effects of toluene on the brain white matter. Individuals with chronic inhalant abuse involving toluene, documented by gas chromatographic analyses demonstrating high concentrations of this solvent in inhaled spray paint fumes, were found to have variable degrees of white matter damage, even on the early MRI scanners with low field strength of .35 T.[19–21] One of the first observations was loss of gray–white matter differentiation, and soon the appearance of periventricular white matter hyperintensity was appreciated. As these changes were invariably diffuse, a widespread effect on white matter was noted (**Fig. 1**). Atrophy of the cerebrum, cerebellum, and brain stem was seen to develop in parallel with these white matter abnormalities. Neurophysiological studies were also consistent with white

Table 2
Clinical, neuroimaging, and neuropathological features of toluene leukoencephalopathy

Dementia	Elemental Neurologic Deficits	MRI Findings	Neuropathology
Apathy and inattention	Cerebellar ataxia, axial, and appendicular	Cerebral, cerebellar, and brain stem atrophy	Diffuse cerebral white matter pallor with normal cortex
Memory impairment	Cranial nerve signs: nystagmus, optic neuropathy, anosmia, hearing loss, ocular flutter, and opsoclonus	Lateral, third, and fourth ventricular enlargement	Sparing of white matter axons until late in the course
Visuospatial dysfunction	Spasticity	Loss of gray–white matter differentiation	Periventricular gliosis
Preserved language	Dysarthria	Periventricular hyperintensity	No inflammatory or vascular change

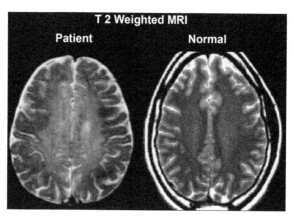

Fig. 1. Axial T2 weighted MRI of a chronic toluene abuser and a normal individual. The scan on the left shows diffuse hyperintensity of the cerebral white matter consistent with widespread myelin injury. (*From* Arciniegas DB, Anderson CA, Filley CM. Behavioral neurology & neuropsychiatry. New York: Cambridge University Press; 2013. p. 425; with permission.)

matter involvement, as brain stem-evoked response testing disclosed abnormal results in toluene abusers.[19] Clinically, various neurologic deficits were identified, including cerebellar ataxia, various cranial nerve signs, spasticity, and dysarthria, but the most disabling of all was dementia.[18] This syndrome was characterized as featuring apathy, inattention, memory loss, and visuospatial dysfunction in the absence of significant aphasia.[18] Further study of this syndrome disclosed 2 key points: that the severity of dementia was correlated not only with the degree of white matter involvement on MRI, but also with the estimated duration of toluene abuse.[22]

Supporting these clinical observations, autopsy reports of toluene abusers demonstrated that cerebral white matter and cerebellar white matter were primarily affected, with normal cortical gray matter, and sparing of axons within white matter until late in the course.[23–25] The corpus callosum, the largest brain white matter tract, was found to be severely affected.[24,26] These reports came mainly from abusers of spray paint[23,24] and glue.[25] One patient came to autopsy after fatal cardiac arrhythmia, presumably induced by stress, which is known to sensitize the myocardium to epinephrine.[23] Inflammatory and vascular alterations were not seen, differentiating this disorder from demyelinative or immune-mediated neuropathology, and from cerebrovascular disease. A direct toxic effect of toluene on myelin came to be suspected, perhaps involving free radical-induced lipid peroxidation, although the pathophysiology of the injury remains obscure.[26] With further study, the predilection of toluene for the brain white matter became increasingly apparent,[26,27] and subsequently, more comprehensive clinical[28] and neuropathological[29] studies added more data confirming that toluene is the major agent in inhalant abusers causing dementia as a result of white matter involvement. Taken together, these observations provided substantial support for toluene being a white matter toxin that specifically targets myelin within brain regions subserving cognition.

From a neurobehavioral perspective, the proposed syndrome of white matter dementia[30] gained strong validation as the emerging data from toluene abuse corroborated observations of dementia resulting from many other white matter disorders. Whereas the most familiar form of dementia is Alzheimer disease, related to primary neuropathology in the cerebral cortex, damage in other brain regions can also produce dementia, and several white matter disorders can prove responsible.[6,30,31] The profile of cognitive deficits listed in **Table 2** is consistent with those encountered in patents with other white matter disorders,[6,30,31] leading to the idea that white matter is an important contributor to the human cognitive repertoire. While this notion may seem at variance with the prevailing neuroscientific emphasis on the cerebral cortex as the mediator of human cognition, recent data demonstrating that human prefrontal white matter has enlarged over the course of evolution even more than gray matter[32] suggest that a strictly corticocentric[33] perspective is too limited. White matter is indeed important for normal cognition, and whereas more study is needed, toluene leukoencephalopathy has proven to be a reliable example of white matter dementia,[6,22,26,30,31] as the selective white matter injury produced by this solvent has become increasingly well established.

PROGNOSIS AND TREATMENT OF INHALANT ABUSE

The management of toluene and other inhalant abuse involves an understanding of both the prognosis of those who are affected and the treatment of this form of substance abuse. Unfortunately, little is known of either topic. For those individuals who do achieve abstinence from inhalant abuse, limited data suggest that some degree of recovery can occur, but much work is needed to establish more knowledge of this area.[34] As follow-up study of abusers is often difficult, most studies are cross-sectional, and few longitudinal data are available; preliminary observations indicate that clinical improvement may be more apparent than resolution of MRI white matter abnormalities.[18,19] One factor influencing the reversibility of white matter changes is likely to be the duration of exposure, as accidental toluene exposure over 6 to 8 months in an otherwise normal adult was followed by cognitive recovery and substantial MRI improvement,[35] whereas longer exposure durations may permit less recoverability.[34] Treatment of inhalant abuse has not been extensively studied, but the similarity of this disorder to other forms of substance abuse implicating dopaminergic transmission illustrates the challenge facing implementation of effective strategies. Like other drugs of abuse, toluene appears to activate the reward system mediated by dopaminergic transmission in the ventral tegmental area and the nucleus accumbens.[36] Prevention has been attempted, with computer-delivered intervention shown to reduce inhalant use in adolescent girls.[1] Efforts to reduce the retail sale of inhalants have been proposed, as has the proposal of adding bittering agents to legally available inhalants.[1] Pharmacotherapy and psychosocial intervention may also help, although few data have been gathered to guide these treatments.[1] One behaviorally oriented program treating adolescent boys noted antisocial traits both before and after 2 years of treatment,[37] confirming the often noted comorbidity of psychiatric disorders and inhalant abuse.[1,16] Treatment programs for inhalant abuse are rare in the United States,[1] and a recent Cochrane review found no adequate studies of treatment and could offer no recommendations.[38]

TOLUENE ABUSE AS A MODEL OF TOXIC LEUKOENCEPHALOPATHY

From a research perspective, toluene abuse offers an instructive model of toxic leukoencephalopathy. Although it cannot be assumed that toluene abusers always confine themselves to a single intoxicant, evidence from the human literature is mounting to document the role of this highly lipophilic solvent in producing direct damage to brain myelin with prominent cognitive sequelae. In addition to the many studies using conventional MRI,[19–22] more advanced neuroimaging has also shown white matter abnormalities. Magnetic resonance spectroscopy of toluene abusers, for example, has disclosed low n-acetyl aspartate, suggesting axonopathy, and elevated myoinositol, consistent with gliosis, in the cerebral and cerebellar white matter that were not found in the thalamus,[39] and preliminary studies with diffusion tensor imaging (DTI) have found reduced fractional anisotropy in the temporal lobe white matter and corpus callosum of inhalant abusers.[40] Experimental studies have also been consistent with this line of inquiry. In keeping with its high lipid solubility, toluene is preferentially taken up in lipid-rich regions of the brains of exposed rats,[41] and is least concentrated in the hippocampus and cerebral cortex.[42] Moreover, rats exposed to toluene have white matter abnormalities on DTI and behavioral evidence of selective cognitive dysfunction without concomitant motor impairment.[43] Some recovery has been documented in toluene-exposed rats after withdrawal of the toxin,[43,44] offering more data to inform the issue of prognosis. Given the particular vulnerability of the CNS to toxic chemicals, and the high volume of myelin within white matter,[45] toluene abuse offers a useful pathophysiological model, and the syndrome of toluene leukoencephalopathy can be seen as prototypical for all the toxic leukoencephalopathies.[2]

One of the many implications of toluene-induced toxic leukoencephalopathy is that a spectrum of severity can be expected given the widely variable exposure that can occur. Indeed such a continuum of leukotoxicity can be seen with exposure to a wide range of chemicals in many medical and nonmedical settings.[2] However, whereas little doubt exists that intense chronic exposure to inhalants such as toluene (often implying daily use of spray paint for years without respite) can result in leukoencephalopathy, much more uncertainty accompanies the possibility that low-level solvent exposure (as might occur in the workplace) can cause harm to the brain. Many reports have attempted to document cognitive dysfunction related to workplace solvent exposure, but studies of workers exposed to relatively low levels of solvents are complicated by confounds such as multiple simultaneous exposures, the lack of unequivocal measures of toxicity, the presence of other problems such as alcohol abuse and psychiatric disorders, and the issue of secondary gain.[26,46] A detailed recent review of this often contentious issue concluded that no reliable conclusions can be drawn about the presence or absence of long-term nervous system damage related to occupational solvent exposure.[47] More clarity in this area will only come with well-designed studies of individuals at risk using rigorous inclusion and exclusion criteria, careful measurements of exposure, and reliable means of detecting leukotoxicity with sensitive clinical, neuroimaging, and, when available, neuropathological investigation.

A final point relevant to this article is the question of selective vulnerability of the young brain to toluene and other leukotoxins. It is increasingly well established that the brain undergoes a normal developmental trajectory whereby white matter gradually forms postnatally and for many years thereafter, only reaching its full adult volume in midlife, around the age of 45.[31] Thus the brains of adolescents and young adults are far from completely myelinated at the time when inhalant abuse typically begins. The implications of this observation are twofold. First, the incomplete myelination of the young brain may account for the relative lack of impulse control and mature decision making that would prevent or moderate the potentially injurious behavior associated with inhalant abuse.[31,48–50] Second, the brains of young inhalant abusers may sustain a more severe leukotoxic effect precisely because of the underdevelopment of white matter.[31,48–50] As a selective myelin toxin, toluene in particular could have an especially damaging effect on adolescent and young adult white matter because of its specific leuktoxicity.[31,48–50] Thus the increase in antisocial behavior over 2 years of continued inhalant abuse in adolescent boys[37] may mean that immature white matter not only predisposes to this form of substance abuse, but often bears a disproportionate burden of the injury produced by the practice.[31,48–50]

SUMMARY

Inhalant abuse is a poorly understood area within the field of substance abuse, so much so that it has been termed the forgotten epidemic.[1] It is clear that this problem deserves more focused investigation in view of the high prevalence of inhalant use, the potential for addiction to inhalants based on their propensity to activate the brain reward system, the often disastrous medical sequelae that can occur, and the relative paucity of information available on the topic in general. Among the many inhalants to which vulnerable individuals have ready access, toluene has become well recognized as a toxin that specifically targets brain myelin. Toluene abuse offers an excellent model of toxic leukoencephalopathy,[2] as its effects on white matter are demonstrable neuroradiologically and neuropathologically and have important neurobehavioral consequences. Much more needs to be learned, both in terms of the clinical approach to inhalant abuse and in pursuing the contributions of white matter to cognitive function, but the evolving investigation of toluene abuse offers promise for greater understanding of these relatively neglected areas.

REFERENCES

1. Howard MO, Bowen SE, Garland EL, et al. Inhalant use and inhalant use disorders in the United States. Addict Sci Clin Pract 2011;6:18–31.
2. Filley CM, Kleinschmidt-DeMasters BK. Toxic leukoencephalopathy. N Engl J Med 2001;345:425–32.
3. Miller AK, Alston RL, Corsellis JA. Variation with age in the volumes of grey and white matter in the cerebral hemispheres of man: measurements with an image analyzer. Neuropathol Appl Neurobiol 1980;6:119–32.
4. Saver JL. Time is brain-quantified. Stroke 2006;37:263–6.
5. Nolte J. The human brain. 5th edition. St Louis (MO): Mosby; 2002.
6. Filley CM. The behavioral neurology of cerebral white matter. Neurology 1998; 50:1535–40.
7. Aralasmak A, Ulmer JL, Kocak M, et al. Association, commissural, and projection pathways and their functional deficit reported in literature. J Comput Assist Tomogr 2006;30:695–715.
8. Filley CM. White matter: organization and functional relevance. Neuropsychol Rev 2010;20:158–73.
9. Schmahmann JD, Pandya DN. Fiber pathways of the brain. New York: Oxford University Press; 2006.
10. Baumann N, Pham-Dinh D. Biology of oligodendrocyte and myelin in the mammalian nervous system. Physiol Rev 2001;81:871–927.
11. Bennaroch EF. Oligodendrocytes. Susceptibility to injury and involvement in neurologic disease. Neurology 2009;72:1779–85.
12. Turken AU, Whitfield-Gabrieli S, Bammer R, et al. Cognitive speed and the structure of white matter pathways: convergent evidence from normal variation and lesion studies. Neuroimage 2008;42:1032–44.
13. Kochunov P, Coyle T, Lancaster J, et al. Processing speed is correlated with cerebral health markers in the frontal lobes quantified by neuroimaging. Neuroimage 2010;49:1190–9.
14. Mesulam MM. Large-scale neurocognitive networks and distributed processing for attention, language, and memory. Ann Neurol 1990;28:597–613.
15. Filley CM. White matter and behavioral neurology. Ann N Y Acad Sci 2005;1064: 162–83.
16. Brouette T, Anton R. Clinical review of inhalants. Am J Addict 2001;10:79–94.

17. Grabski DA. Toluene sniffing producing cerebellar degeneration. Am J Psychiatry 1961;118:461–2.
18. Hormes JT, Filley CM, Rosenberg NL. Neurologic sequelae of chronic solvent vapor abuse. Neurology 1986;36:698–702.
19. Rosenberg NL, Spitz MC, Filley CM, et al. Central nervous system effects of chronic toluene abuse—clinical, brainstem evoked response and magnetic resonance imaging studies. Neurotoxicol Teratol 1988;10:489–95.
20. Yamanouchi N, Okada S, Kodama K, et al. White matter changes caused by chronic solvent abuse. AJNR Am J Neuroradiol 1995;16:1643–9.
21. Aydin K, Sencer S, Demir T, et al. Cranial MR findings in chronic toluene abuse by inhalation. AJNR Am J Neuroradiol 2002;23:1173–9.
22. Filley CM, Heaton RK, Rosenberg NL. White matter dementia in chronic toluene abuse. Neurology 1990;40:532–4.
23. Rosenberg NK, Kleinschmidt-DeMasters BK, Davis KA, et al. Toluene abuse causes diffuse central nervous system white matter changes. Ann Neurol 1988;23:611–4.
24. Kornfeld M, Moser AB, Moser HW, et al. Solvent vapor abuse leukoencephalopathy. Comparison to adrenoleukodystrophy. J Neuropathol Exp Neurol 1994;53:389–98.
25. Marulanda N, Colegial C. Neurotoxicity of solvents in brain of glue abusers. Environ Toxicol Pharmacol 2005;19:671–5.
26. Filley CM, Halliday W, Kleinschmidt-DeMasters BK. The effects of toluene on the central nervous system. J Neuropathol Exp Neurol 2004;63:1–12.
27. Rosenberg NL, Grigsby J, Dreisbach J, et al. Neuropsychologic impairment and MRI abnormalities associated with chronic solvent abuse. J Toxicol Clin Toxicol 2002;40:21–34.
28. Yücel M, Takagi M, Walterfang M, et al. Toluene misuse and long-term harms: a systematic review of the neuropsychological and neuroimaging literature. Neurosci Biobehav Rev 2008;32:910–26.
29. Al-Hajri Z, Del Bigio MR. Brain damage in a large cohort of solvent abusers. Acta Neuropathol 2010;119:435–45.
30. Filley CM, Franklin GM, Heaton RK, et al. White matter dementia. Clinical disorders and implications. Neuropsychiatry Neuropsychol Behav Neurol 1988;1:239–54.
31. Filley CM. The behvavioral neurology of white matter. 2nd edition. New York: Oxford University Press; 2012.
32. Schoenemann PT, Sheehan MJ, Glotzer LD. Prefrontal white matter volume is disproportionately larger in humans than in other primates. Nat Neurosci 2005;8:242–52.
33. Parvizi J. Corticocentric myopia: old bias in new cognitive sciences. Trends Cogn Sci 2009;13:354–9.
34. Takagi M, Lubman DI, Yücel M. Solvent-induced leukoencephalopathy: a disorder of adolescence? Subst Use Misuse 2011;46(Suppl 1):95–8.
35. Qureshi SU, Blanchette AR, Jawaid A, et al. Reversible leukoencephalopathy due to chronic unintentional exposure to toluene. Can J Neurol Sci 2009;36:388–9.
36. Lubman DI, Yücel M, Lawrence AJ. Inhalant abuse among adolescents: neurobiological considerations. Br J Pharmacol 2008;154:316–26.
37. Sakai JT, Mikulich-Gilbertson SK, Crowley TJ. Adolescent inhalant use among male patients in treatment for substance and behavior problems: two-year outcome. Am J Drug Alcohol Abuse 2006;32:29–40.

38. Konghom S, Verachai V, Srisurapanont M, et al. Treatment for inhalant dependence and abuse. Cochrane Database Syst Rev 2010;(12):CD007537.
39. Aydin K, Sencer S, Ogel K, et al. Single-voxel proton MR spectroscopy in toluene abuse. Magn Reson Imaging 2003;21:777–85.
40. Yücel M, Zalesky A, Takagi MJ, et al. White-matter abnormalities in adolescents with long-term inhalant and cannabis use: a diffusion magnetic resonance imaging study. J Psychiatry Neurosci 2010;35:409–12.
41. Gospe SM, Calaban MJ. Central nervous system distribution of inhaled toluene. Fundam Appl Toxicol 1988;11:540–5.
42. Ameno K, Kiriu T, Fuke C, et al. Regional brain distribution of toluene in rats and in a human autopsy. Arch Toxicol 1992;66:153–6.
43. Duncan JR, Dick AL, Egan G, et al. Adolescent toluene inhalation in rats affects white matter maturation with the potential for recovery following abstinence. PLoS One 2012;7:e44790.
44. Schiffer WK, Lee DE, Alexoff DL, et al. Metabolic correlates of toluene abuse: decline and recovery of function in adolescent animals. Psychopharmacology 2006;186:159–67.
45. Harris JB, Blain PG. Neurotoxicology: what the neurologist needs to know. J Neurol Neurosurg Psychiatry 2004;75(Suppl 3):iii29–34.
46. Schaumburg HH, Albers JW. Pseudoneurotoxic disease. Neurology 2005;62:22–6.
47. Ridgway P, Nixon TE, Leach JP. Occupational exposure to organic solvents and long-term nervous system damage detectable by brain imaging, neurophysiology or histopathology. Food Chem Toxicol 2003;41:153–87.
48. Kumar A, Cook IA. White matter injury, neural connectivity and the pathophysiology of psychiatric disorders. Dev Neurosci 2002;24:255–61.
49. Bartzokis G. Brain myelination in prevalent neuropsychiatric developmental disorders: primary and comorbid addiction. Adolesc Psychiatry 2005;29:55–96.
50. Fields RD. White matter in learning, cognition, and psychiatric disorders. Trends Neurosci 2008;31:361–70.

Index

Note: Page numbers of article titles are in **boldface** type.

Psychiatr Clin N Am 36 (2013) 303–307
http://dx.doi.org/10.1016/S0193-953X(13)00055-5
0193-953X/13/$ – see front matter © 2013 Elsevier Inc. All rights reserved.

psych.theclinics.com

Moving?

Make sure your subscription moves with you!

To notify us of your new address, find your **Clinics Account Number** (located on your mailing label above your name), and contact customer service at:

Email: journalscustomerservice-usa@elsevier.com

800-654-2452 (subscribers in the U.S. & Canada)
314-447-8871 (subscribers outside of the U.S. & Canada)

Fax number: 314-447-8029

Elsevier Health Sciences Division
Subscription Customer Service
3251 Riverport Lane
Maryland Heights, MO 63043

Printed and bound by CPI Group (UK) Ltd, Croydon, CR0 4YY

03/10/2024

01040441-0010